ONE CRAZY BROCCOLI!

BROCCOLI!

— Compiled by **CHRISTINE MARMOY** —

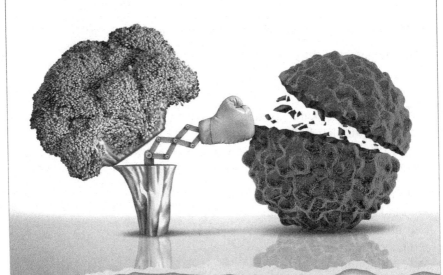

My Body is Smarter than My Disease

CM Publisher
c/o Marketing for Coach, Ltd
Second Floor
6th London Street
W2 1HR London (UK)

www.cm-publisher.com
info@cm-publisher.com

ISBN: 978-0-9929876-8-8

Published in UK, Europe, US and Canada

Book Cover: Csernik Előd

Inside Layout: Csernik Előd

Maureen:

To your health!

Stacy Cromwell

Table of Contents

Disclaimer

Every word in this book is based on the personal experience, anecdotal evidence and expertise of the various authors who have participated in the co-creation of this book.

Although all those involved made every reasonable attempt to achieve complete accuracy in the content shared in this book, neither I, Christine Marmoy, nor my publishing company, CM Publisher, assume any responsibility for errors or omissions. You should only use this information as you see fit and at your own risk. Your situation may not be ideally suited to the examples shared within the following pages and therefore as the reader, you are solely responsible for how you use the information available to you.

Most of the co-authors are not doctors, dieticians or fitness trainers; therefore please seek professional expertise in these areas. All the information we share is what we have tested on ourselves and the results we obtained.

Nothing in this book is intended to replace medical advice and is in no way a magic trick to regain health without having to make drastic changes. The results achieved by each person may well vary.

Thank You

This book will be the first in a long series, I sure hope so. It has been the easiest book we have organized and published so far, which I take as another strong sign from the Universe. And for the precious pages you are holding in your hands right now, I have many people to thank, people I'm so grateful to have in my life, to call my team or to consider as friends.

First of all, I'd like to thank the Universe. Although I already do it every day, I never fully acknowledge its help publicly. Before I was in the midst of a heavy brain fog brought on by new health challenges as you'll discover in my story, I asked the Universe a few months ago to show me how to reunite again a few passions of mine....the Universe answered me with strength and conviction. I got sick and then found my way! Thanks again for knocking me down every time; it seems like it's the only way I learn.

Next, I'd like to thank all the co-authors who shared their stories with such candor and openness. For some of them it was not an easy task. But they did it, and I'm so proud of each and every one of them. I interviewed every person sharing their story in this book, I asked them about their story, I asked them about their values and their mission. I'm so fortunate to have met them all. Yet again, another chance situation through divine intervention. After having spoken with every one of them, I can assure you that they are all genuine, honest and amazingly loving people. They truly care! Nowadays it's so hard to find people who really care from the depth of their heart.

With help from the Universe I was able to gather together a wonderful group of people to whom I'll always be grateful. I can vouch for all of them, for their quality of heart but also for their dedication in their respective areas of expertise. You can trust them as much as I do.

Then, not least of all, I would like to thank my team who are always on the ready to jump on any new idea I throw at them. As usual, thank you to Jane Bell, my Executive Assistant on the Coaching & Success side of my business who is always willing to help in any capacity she can, above and beyond the call of duty. Another special thank you to Claudia Ramos, our new strong pillar, my Executive/Personal Assistant on the Raw & More side. She knows how to navigate the flux of change and handle just about anything I delegate to her. For the past year she has been a strong shoulder on which I was able to fully lean, hence the reason she won the title of "Angel". This beautiful book would not have gone to print without the professionalism and the quality of work of my amazing designer, Előd Csernik, who will be a 'Daddy' by the time he receives this book. Congratulations, Elod, you'll be a terrific father.

Last but not least, thank you to my family. You are as crazy as before if not more, and I love you just the way you are. A special thank you goes to my husband, Pascal, who is willing to change many things, just because he loves me. Thank you to my little ball of love, Mathys, who is my teacher and my accomplice. You challenge me every day to go further, to find new recipes to eat, to find new ways to live allergy free.

Thank you, my dear readers, because without you, these stories would only be just that—stories. Now they become messages, they become letters of hope, of joy, of possibility for you and for everyone you know...... and all thanks to each and every one of you.

Introduction

When I first got the idea for this book, I was in the midst of a heavy brain fog, sick beyond anything I had ever experienced before and desperately worried because this time I wasn't the only one feeling really ill. My 6 year old was going through the same ordeal, even if his symptoms were slightly different. I didn't know what to do and I was in a total panic (at least, when I had the strength!) because most of the time I could barely get out of bed....and I couldn't take care of my baby who was feeling just as bad.

Then one evening I was looking for a book, a testimonial from a mom who had gone through what I was experiencing and who could have helped me. I wanted to know what others had done before me to regain their health and to ensure it never happened again. Yet that night I couldn't find it. Maybe that book does exist somewhere, but I didn't find it....the brain fog could have been to blame.

That is when it occurred to me: You have a publishing company, why don't you publish that book yourself?

I had been looking for a way to combine my business—the publishing of books as a marketing tool—with my all-time passion for food, health and fitness. I didn't connect the dots right away; I had to wait until the next morning when talking with a friend who actually turned round and said: wow that makes total sense, this is so you! And there you have it, One Crazy Broccoli was born.

My goal with this book was to bring together a wide range of people from different backgrounds, walks of life, experiences, statuses, careers, ethnicities and spiritual practices in order to ensure that this book would cover as much ground as possible while appealing to as many readers as possible.

My vision, and the one shared by all the co-authors participating in this book, is to allow One Crazy Broccoli to become your favorite book—the one you keep on your bedside table—as a written guide which you are drawn to whenever your state of health challenges you, whenever you feel discouraged, whenever you start saying to yourself: "Whatever!" The one book you want to offer to your loved ones who may also be suffering in their own body.

However, my vision was way short of what this book ended up becoming. It's a real tribute, a prayer with many verses, a compass for those who are lost, a fluffy pillow for those who need to rest their weary heads, a warm blanket for those who feel cold, a shoulder to lean on, a guide with many different voices and many different faces. But more importantly than all that, it is tangible proof offered to you. A proof of your power, of what you are capable of doing right now, in this moment, exactly where you are. You have the power to change your health and to recover joy and fulfillment.

Each word is a loving kiss on your wounds, each line is a song emanating directly from the co-authors' hearts, each chapter is a testimonial of strength, courage, power and willingness in the face of adversity. Each story is a heart-crushing testament to the fact that you too can learn how to navigate your way round the rocks, across the currents and the fallen branches that sometimes get strewn across the river that represents the flow of life.

What astounded me most of all when I read the full manuscript is that every single Soul in this book was willing to share how much in the dark they once were, how fearful and panic stricken they were, how little they knew before embarking on this amazing wave of change for the greater good, for saving and recovering their life.

Each chapter in this book brought tears to my eyes, as well as a smile to my face—I even found myself nodding in agreement more than once, as I'm sure you'll do as well. Sure enough, you'll most likely recognize yourself in the lines and pages that follow even if it's not exactly your story, just as much as I found myself on certain occasions.

When we first ventured out on this project, I asked all the wonderful co-authors who contributed to this masterpiece to be as honest as possible and to give a part of themselves to you. I also asked them to relate their story but to pay particular attention to the message they shared. I invited them to recount in great detail what they did to be able to change their health around and to recover the life they have today. I strongly believe in the quote that says: "What you focus on expands". Therefore, I wanted all of them to focus on the positive in order to lead you toward the positive as well, along with sharing pertinent and practical information that you could implement right away.

They truly over-delivered on that request! Reading this book will propel you into an adventurous journey inside: You will reconnect with certain feelings you thought were gone forever and out of reach, you will recall episodes in your own life and suddenly a light will appear to illuminate the darkness you may have in your mind, and you will understand and embrace the power of forgiveness and acceptance. You will find the strength to tackle your health from many different angles and to tap into that huge ocean of wisdom that makes life flow.

This flow can only truly be seen when we are aligned; it is always there, in its tranquility as well as in its strength as a rock. However, most of us (myself included!) spend the majority of our life blindfold in the face of this evidence! Until years later, this same evidence comes and knocks us down with so much force that we cannot deny it, we cannot keep our eyes shut, we need to wake up and act to live or sleep to die.

Nevertheless, it exists, and its power is unquestionable and undeniable.

The only question I may ask of you is: Are you ready? Are you ready to open your mind to the possibility that you too can make a complete

U-turn in your health as you know it right now in order to allow yourself to step into your own power and gain access to healing.

Between the lines, this book conveys a few messages. First and foremost, I wish from the bottom of my heart that you'll find within these stories some pearls of wisdom that you'll be moved to implement until good health returns.

Sadly, I've realized when talking with many people over the course of a year, that some of them now feel guilty for their poor health. They understand that it is their own fault and they are the problem causing the situation in which they undoubtedly find themselves in at this very moment. I so wish this book will help them come to terms and find peace with this thought. Many of us fell sick through lack of knowledge; yes, we are responsible but that doesn't mean we are guilty! Once you are aware, you can save the situation, you can change what must be changed and at anytime you can transform yourself. The same power you used to get sick can also be used to get you healthy. And no matter what you do or think, this power is always there nestled in the core of your being.

My hope for this book is not only to help those struggling with serious health conditions. I also hope to help those who aren't sick, those who are concerned about their health and want to make sure that whatever they do is the right thing for their body.

This book can be a cure as much as a preventive guide. It's up to you, the reader.

Think of this book as a small step toward achieving that goal, to help you refocus on what is important and help you understand how to become the healer in your own life.

This book has been put together so it is easy to read. Each story is easy to relate to, each concept is easy to grasp. The difficulty will lie in your own ability to push away the self-imposed limits that you placed on yourself a long time ago and to facilitate the emergence of what is trying to make its way through your heart by the manifestation of everything that is going wrong in your life right now.

Feel free to read one chapter at a time, or jump to the story that is most relevant to your own situation, or read the entire book in one day. It's entirely up to you how you wish to use it, but you will undoubtedly end up reading it all!

Don't let fear overcome you into a forced status quo. Reclaim your liberty. Take control of your own freedom and make the decision that what matters most in life for you right now—is YOU.

CHAPTER 1

HOW TO RECOVER FROM SEXUAL VIOLENCE

By Claire Higgins

I remember the morning after. I remember the year. But I can't tell you which day or month it was. Was it June? Was it July? There are some details my mind has blocked out forever.

I remember waking up to the sound of his movements in the bedroom. I lay there in my teenage single bed, eyes squeezed shut, still not able to move. My body had been frozen in the same position for hours, flat on my back, face up to the ceiling.

I had floated up to the dimmer light on the upper right hand wall not long after he had climbed into my bed. Because I was no longer there, I didn't feel the searing pain between my legs or the crushing weight on my chest that arrived next.

He left quietly, and only then did I begin to relax. At some point I got up and showered. I may have drunk a glass of water. Before the morning ended, he called me.

"I'm sorry for last night," he said.

"It doesn't matter," I responded.

And that was that. With those three words, I had just negated my self-worth for the next fifteen years. A light inside of me had gone out, and it would take another lifetime to get it back.

A few months after that fateful night, the skin on my face erupted in angry, red welts. It was as if my body was trying to say what I could not. At night, they itched so intensely that even gloves couldn't stop my hands from clawing my skin to pieces.

Soon, the skin became just as torn and damaged as the rest of me. The red turned to fiery orange. Each morning, I wept as I washed my face. I soon learned that the skin on my face could no longer tolerate water or exposure to sun, so I used a non-rinse facial cleanser, put SPF 50 on my face, and began to spend more time indoors.

Until that moment, I had been a strong swimmer and outdoors girl, competing regularly in swimming galas. I lived across the road from the beach, my second home, and my bookshelf was covered with medals, trophies, and certificates. I was known for being athletic and bold, but after the event, I began to withdraw.

I found a refuge in art and writing music. I stopped socializing with friends and, instead, locked myself up in my bedroom. There, I had my art desk and piano. They took some of the pain away as I poured my heart out into my creative endeavors.

I couldn't tell anyone what had happened. How could I explain that my body had betrayed me and froze the instant he attacked me? I was also a Karate student and, by then, I had been training for almost three years. I held a purple belt, but that belt hadn't protected me when I needed it most.

Over the years, the eczema spread from my face to my arms and legs. I spent many hours bandaging different parts of my body several times a day. My weight plummeted as I restricted my food intake. By the time I passed my black belt test in Karate at the age of 20, my face was pale and gaunt.

One morning, my Sensei dragged me to the mirror in our training dojo, or hall, and pointed out the black circles under my eyes.

"You're not eating!" he yelled at me.

That was the day I started wearing concealer under my eyes. I thought if I could better hide the pain, it would go away. But it didn't.

It took me many years to understand just how much teenage sexual violence had affected my life. On reflection, I can see how it drove me into politics and over a decade of humanitarian work. There, I witnessed some of the world's worst atrocities, including rape and other forms of sexual violence.

Through my work, I became a strong advocate for the protection of others, but inwardly, I had yet to heal and protect myself. Eventually, at twenty-nine, I could no longer deny how broken I felt inside. It was then that I made a very conscious decision to turn my life around and put my own healing process first.

That year, I trained as a Yoga teacher to learn more about healing and the body. Within months, I left an abusive marriage. At thirty-two, after my divorce came through, I entered two years of therapy.

By then, I was working in refugee camps in a war zone and had to do most of my therapy on Skype. It wasn't easy to do this long distance, but I didn't have another option, and I wasn't about to backtrack on my commitment to heal myself.

In my free time, I taught Yoga to women affected by stress, trauma, and violence. The following year, I trained as a health coach to better understand the link between violence and health. This led me to coach a team of doctors and nurses through a health community outreach strategy for over a million refugees affected by war.

At thirty-four, I finally broke nineteen years of silence and told everyone I knew the story of sexual violence that I had lived. I returned to my Karate training and made a choice never to give up on myself again. I had learned how to be there for myself as well as others

At thirty-six, I am now a strong and healthy black belt. My skin is clear and I can't remember the last time I experienced an eczema outbreak. The shame of my teenage sexual violence is long gone.

I believe that the potential for violence of any kind, including sexual, increases when we stop communicating with ourselves and each other. It's one of the reasons why I'm now a professionally trained coach and communications specialist.

When we don't say what matters and when we don't express how we truly feel, our emotions can get stuck inside of us. This only leads to more pain and, often, poor decision-making. It increases the potential for further conflict inside and around us and, eventually, this can lead to more violence.

If there is anything I have learned over the past twenty-one years, it is that each of us has a unique timing and way for healing. There are as many healing paths from sexual violence as there are people affected, and no one way is the "right" way. However, there are basic building blocks that we can all draw from in our recovery.

At the top of the list are getting adequate sleep, remembering to breathe, and taking time to rest. This is because the first casualty of sexual violence and trauma is the nervous system. This is our internal communications network. It passes information from one part of our body to another through the connection of nerves. When a shock or trauma hits, this network can start to malfunction. When unresolved stress becomes greater than what we can inwardly handle, the network can even go down. In everyday terms, we call this burnout or a nervous breakdown.

Yoga was the first healing mechanism that worked for me. It is, by far, one of the most effective practices I know of that can heal and repair a damaged nervous system. Gentle forms of Yoga that prioritize breathing exercises, relaxation, and mental rest can go a long way in a sexual trauma survivor's recovery.

If you struggle with getting a good night's sleep, gentle Yoga has the added benefit of preparing your mind and body to turn inwards. A short and silent meditation practice of five to ten minutes can encourage more inner quiet and peace.

Yet healing is not only about fostering peace. Sometimes it is about getting very, very angry with what was done to us. We absolutely need to pass through this phase of anger and possibly rage if we are to truly be at peace within ourselves. If we do not allow space for such expression, we run the risk of further repressing our pain.

Accessing our deepest emotions happens when we bring more of our body into our healing journey. As Bessel Van Der Kolk, a trauma expert, says, "Our bodies keep the score." They remember everything that has happened to us, including memories of sexual trauma.

On my healing journey, I worked first with a **Dance Movement Psychotherapist** who led me through verbal and non-verbal therapy. Later, I worked with a **Clinical Psychologist and Somatic Experiencing (SE) Practitioner**. SE is a form of bodily-oriented trauma therapy developed by Dr. Peter Levine.

Parallel to this, I learned how to nourish my body through **food and nutrition**. Through my **Health Coach Training**, I learned to identify foods that supported my nervous system, which had been exposed to so much post-traumatic stress. I focused on eating plenty of essential fatty acids, which fortified my skin and soothed my nerves.

After more than a decade of vegetarianism, I began eating fish, chicken, and meat again. The **extra protein** helped me to regain a healthy weight and muscle tone. It also stabilized my energy levels throughout the day, which post-traumatic stress had affected for years. This helped me to sustain my workouts, and gradually, my body became stronger, as well as my mind.

Developing a **spiritual practice** when I came out of therapy eased the emotional transition for me. I found a group of like-minded women from all ages and walks of life and a wise woman who taught me the healing powers of establishing daily rituals and disciplines like meditation, breathing, movement, journaling, and regularly turning inwards.

Coaching was also an essential healing mechanism as it helped me to clarify and crystallize my learning process. It provided me with essential tools and practical life skills to translate what I was learning into practice. It held me accountable and provided a container in which I truly believed I could do anything I set my heart to.

Several years into my healing journey, I broke my silence through **writing**, first via weekly blogging, which I kept up for two years, and later, through a book on how to journey beyond violence, conflict, stress, trauma, and adversity.

While the blogging was about my story, the book was about me in relation to others who had experienced adversities such as cancer, natural disasters, imprisonment, and getting shot. I used Carl Jung's framework of the Archetypes to help us **reach out and relate** to each other. This marked another turning point in my recovery, the ability to provide space for others to tell their story.

Perhaps the greatest gift that has come out of healing has been a renewed desire to create. I paint in my free time and find it gives me much joy and peace. With that has come the desire to love from a whole and healthy place. Sexual violence can shatter a woman's ability to feel safe in relationships. Once she is healed, it is easier to relax and trust that life can and will be good.

RESOURCES

Dance Movement Psychotherapy: **www.admt.org.uk**

Somatic Experiencing: **www.traumahealing.org**

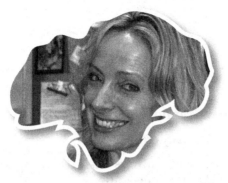

Tracy Cromwell

Certified Integrative Nutrition Health Coach / Anti-Aging Consultant

Since 2009, Tracy has been helping clients age "well" by focusing on whole nutrition, antioxidants and gene expression science to increase energy and vitality support for the body as well as recommending non-surgical skin treatments and products that help the skin fend off the visible signs of aging.

Diagnosed as pre-diabetic in 2006, Tracy had to start making better lifestyle choices. A yo-yo dieter most of her life, although this diagnoses was frustrating it put her on a solid path to wellness. After trial and error, she was able to make necessary lifestyle changes and is no longer pre-diabetic. At 48, she feels healthy and strong taking on century bike rides and staying fit. She is making the right food choices for her body. This experience compelled her to go back to school so that she could add complete holistic & integrative health coaching programs to her anti-aging business. Tracy received her training from the Institute for Integrative Nutrition, where she trained in more than 100 dietary theories and studied a variety of practical lifestyle coaching methods. She now helps clients create a completely personalized "roadmap to health" that suits their unique body, lifestyle, preferences, and goals.

Contact Tracy:

www.innovationsinantiaging.com

www.legacycaring.com/members/innovationsinantiaging

www.innovationsinantiaging.blogspot.com

✉ tracycromwell@innovationsinantiaging.com

f facebook.com/tracy.cromwell

f facebook.com/Innovations-In-Anti-Aging-
LLC-226175734092079/timeline/

🐦 @tracycromwell

in linkedin.com/in/tracycromwell

CHAPTER 2

CHANGING MY STARS

By Tracy Cromwell

I was given the opportunity of a lifetime, an opportunity to change my stars. I was diagnosed pre-diabetic by my doctor. I stood tall and chose to walk the road to wellness, not the road to chronic disease.

It has been so interesting to look back on my life and think about how I "felt" throughout it. As far back as childhood, I recall having an incredibly high level of anxiety. I also recall not feeling very well most of the time. It was a normal day to be pretty distressed, yet lethargic combined with a very low threshold for exertion.

My journey to wellness was riddled with a great deal of failure. I had been a "yo-yo" dieter since my high school years. Food was my comfort and my nemesis. You see, I saw myself as never "good enough." I felt unworthy. I was not perfect like other people. I was far from deserving of my life's dreams. It was always someone else's turn before mine. "Don't shine too brightly Tracy," I would think to myself, "who are you to be anything." A constant inner struggle that I didn't understand as an adult, let alone as a child, was always tormenting me.

I know today that many of my emotional challenges were actually triggered by my diet. My diet was making me sick. My diet would make my stomach hurt and my heart race, thus giving me feelings of anxiety and distress. My diet was wreaking havoc on my body and mind.

I would have a meal then feel sick. I would then try to eat something else in an attempt to feel better. It became a vicious cycle: gaining weight, dieting, gaining weight, dieting. I thought it was normal to feel this way so I didn't think to tell anyone.

One of my favorite foods since childhood is popcorn. We had homemade popcorn almost every night. I now know popcorn was one of the main reasons I woke up feeling lethargic and nauseated. For breakfast, my mother would send me off to school with a good breakfast. Oatmeal was a staple, but it always made me feel nauseated. Add this to my popcorn hangover and I dreaded eating breakfast. Mom was wonderful and tried various other options, but it was difficult to find something that worked. I recall in 5th grade going to school feeling anxious and ill, getting diarrhea, being sent to the office with terrible stomach cramps, and being sent home, just to have this repeat again and again. It was eventually determined that I was not ill. I was having anxiety issues that I would have to grow out of. No one knew to look at my food as the possible instigator. It was 1977.

My first weight loss "diet" was at age 17, followed by another diet at age 19 (the Pay-Day-Candy-Bar-for-Lunch Diet). Eventually, I did lose weight and felt pretty good about my size, but I still had immense anxiety. In 1994, I became obsessed with step aerobics. I also started taking fat burning pills which were very harmful. I did all I could to stay a "healthy" weight. Every day I beat myself up doing step aerobics at the highest level while utilizing hand weights to make the workout even more difficult. I looked great! I looked fit! Inside, I was a disaster. I saw this lifestyle as my ONLY way to keep the weight off. If I didn't kill myself with the aerobics, I would start putting the fat back on. One day, I just got tired. I recall it vividly. I stopped step aerobics and never did it again. My jeans started to get tighter; the weight came back.

By my early 40's, I had "yo-yoed" many times. I had a great deal of stress and a knee injury, was working long hours, wasn't exercising, and was enjoying too much wine and chocolate, and it all got me into trouble. I was 30 lbs over-weight, unhappy, and giving up. I recall wishing I had appreciated my body a long time ago instead of hating it. I bought into the "everyone has this happen as they age" mentality. Gradually, I started to notice that I was often very thirsty and always having to run to the restroom. It was definitely a different "kind" of thirst and definitely a different kind of "potty urge." I went in for my annual physical and was told that I was pre-diabetic. This was yet another reason to hate my body and add to the high frustration I already had with myself. Why had I allowed this to happen? I was a bad person. Yet, at the same time, a small voice started speaking to me. "This could be your chance." Maybe I could get my body back and do it the right way, whatever that was. Maybe I could really lose the weight I had gained. Could I feel better, feel strong? Just maybe I could. I finally had a "real" reason to figure out what was going on with my body.

I didn't want to go on yet another "diet." I was tired of dieting. I didn't want to feel deprived. I didn't want to be different from my family, friends, and co-workers. I didn't understand at that time in my life that the food I was eating was actually depriving me of a happy, healthy, and vibrant life. I didn't understand that the food I was eating was actually taking life away from me! I hadn't yet learned to listen to my body. I was still forcing my poor body to accept whatever I blindly put in my mouth and swallowed.

So how did I get myself out of this mess?

My first assignment was minimizing my sugar intake and eliminating refined carbohydrates by switching to whole grains. No problem, right? Not so fast. At home, I had a big pantry full of beautiful white flour, various breakfast cereals, chips, tortilla chips, yummy white penne pasta and white linguine noodles, instant baking mixes, popcorn, white rice, bread, cookies, fruit snacks, crackers, pretzels, etc. I also had two teenagers and a husband at home that liked ALL of those wonderful "foods"! So how was I going to do this?

I started by eliminating breads and pastas. Pasta was very challenging for me. I absolutely LOVE a wonderful al dente pasta noodle smothered with a zesty red marinara or a creamy Alfredo chicken mushroom sauce, then topped with fresh parmesan cheese. What more could a girl ask for? (Well, now I know, a girl can ask for a vibrant, healthy life instead!) I started integrating whole grain pasta with my white pasta. I now substitute spaghetti squash or cauliflower and have eliminated pasta all together.

As time progressed, I began to pay attention to how I *felt* before, during, and after I ate. I finally understood that I did not have to

21

feel sick. I learned to eat "mindfully." If I began to feel sick during or after a meal, I made a mental note of that food and did my best to not eat it again. This has been the biggest lesson and truly one of the greatest reasons I have succeeded at changing my stars. I now "hear" my body.

With some prodding by a friend of mine, I got back on my bicycle. She began by bringing me to spin classes which then led to me riding in The Seattle Tour de Cure, a fund raiser for the American Diabetes Association. I trained for the ride and accomplished 70 miles the first year. I have since ridden 100 miles every year for them. I now crave physical exercise and enjoy cycling and weight training.

Over the past years, I have revised my diet immensely. Please note that I said "years." It didn't happen overnight for me and now it is a consistent, yet fun experiment.

I now "nourish" my body with whole foods and lean proteins, not poison it. I take high quality supplements to get the nutrients lacking in my diet. Although I do not count them, I make sure that my calories have a positive impact and purpose. To get to this point, I had to retrain my brain and work through some serious sugar and refined carbohydrate craving issues. Patience and compassion towards me and my body was vital. Eventually, I learned what my cravings really meant by asking myself questions. Was I thirsty? Did I need fruit? Was I bored or upset?

I now feel blessed by my past life experiences. My journey has led me to invest in myself and in my family's health. It led me to attend The Institute for Integrative Nutrition where I became a Certified Integrative Nutrition Health Coach. I have found my purpose in life. Something that I believe in and knew all this time and never acknowledged. I am meant to help others live a healthy and enriching life. I don't believe I could have fulfilled this purpose without living my past.

We are not meant to be sick. Our bodies are meant to be thriving! By first making a solid commitment, getting out of my own way, then listening mindfully and intently, I can now say at 48 years old, I feel better than I ever have! I am no longer pre-diabetic. It took a scary diagnosis to wake me up and my life will never be the same again!

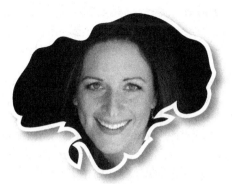

Elicia Miller

Candida Expert, Motivational Speaker, Author, Certified Holistic Health Coach, Inner Child & Journaling Facilitator and Emotional Intuitive

Elicia has guided hundreds to freedom from Candida and emotional chains, but just like any wounded healer, she had to go through her own process first. After a string of abusive relationships (including to herself), multiple addictions, and ongoing physical complaints, she resolved to get free from unwanted symptoms and patterns with relationships and jobs. Frustrated with the lack of results from traditional doctors and therapists, Elicia researched and tried over 50 detox and healing methods. Her journey led her to sell her possessions and spend three years in Thailand, Costa Rica, San Francisco, and Atlanta, working with the best spiritual, ancestral, shamanic, energy, and emotional healers on the planet. As Elicia immersed herself on a path toward physical, mental, and emotional enlightenment, she realized that Candida was more than just symptoms like bloating and yeast infections. Candida was also a manifestation of perfectionism, obsession with outside approval, unresolved trauma, and chronic victim mentality. This newfound understanding of the mind-emotional-body connection gave her freedom and clarity in all aspects of her life. For many years, via Skype, Elicia has been working with people from all over the world who still suffer after wasting time and money on programs that focus solely on diet and supplements.

She created a Candida eCourse as the culmination of 10 years of her expert-level training, personal healing, and research distilled into a guided, step-by-step process to address all aspects of Candida.

Fitting with this collection of Wild Broccoli tales, Elicia's favorite food when she was three years old was broccoli. Elicia is the author of *Detox 101* eBook. She has been interviewed by Wigwam Wellness Festival, Hot & Healthy Podcast, Not Another Diet Summit, Sonic Yogi on Emotional Cleansing and Candida Detox, Suzanne Boothby in *Coming Clean, A Conscious Guide to Food Cleanses,* and featured in *Narrow Escape from an Ordinary Life: A True Story* by Grace G. Payge.

Contact Elicia:

www.eliciamiller.com

415-623-9465

epowerme

elicia@eliciamiller.com

facebook.com/EliciaMillerPage

@eliciammiller

@eliciammiller

pinterest.com/eliciammiller/

youtube.com/detoxworldtour

linkedin.com/in/eliciamiller

CHAPTER 3

CANDIDA AND VICTIMHOOD
By Elicia Miller

Candida defined my life for years. Normally, Candida yeast inhabits the mouth, throat, intestines and urinary tract and is part of a healthy flora that coexists in the lower digestive tract. However, when there is a disturbance in the balance of flora, or a weakening of the host from other causes, it may cause problems and lead to disease.

Such was my story. Candida leached my physical, mental, emotional, and spiritual vibrancy from childhood into early adulthood. I suffered from chronic fatigue, fungal infections, brain fog, bloating and constipation, irritability, sugar and carbohydrate cravings, and many other symptoms associated with Candida. I grew into a struggling, frustrated woman…until I came full circle to discover the root of my symptoms and connect with my greatest truth—that I was more powerful than I'd ever imagined.

YOUR SYMPTOMS ARE A GIFT!

Symptoms are gifts and exist to tell us something. Unfortunately, we often ignore and suppress them, just as I did through parts of my life. I spent thousands of dollars, saw dozens of healers and practitioners, and faithfully followed one diet after another to find the solution to my Candida. All played a part in my healing, either by showing what wasn't the cause or by being a stepping-stone to the ultimate resolution. Everyone's healing journey is unique, but I believe the wisdom garnered from my struggle and story can be life changing to many searching for who they really are beyond Candida.

As a child, I had reoccurring strep throat (which always appeared on my birthday) and found myself taking antibiotics on a regular schedule. Rather than finding the root of my susceptibility to the chronic bacteria, doctors simply recommended I remove my tonsils. By the time I was a young adult, I had advanced from strep throat to reoccurring BV (bacterial vaginosis), UTIs (bladder infections) and frequent bouts with the flu, usually after too much drinking and drug use. The treatment for all was, again, antibiotics.

Antibiotics derives from the Greek word *anti* means "against," and the Greek word bios *means "life"* (bacteria are *life* forms). They kill both the good and bad bacteria that live in the gut. So at the end of my treatments, I consistently developed a yeast infection requiring even more drugs to treat. This vicious cycle went on for several years until I found myself in the doctor's office every month. She told me that some women are just more susceptible to BV infections and that I would need to stay on medicine for the rest of my life. Insanity! Finally, after years of ineffective treatment and spending a small fortune on co-pays, I broke down in tears and left that office searching for the root cause.

I knew there was an imbalance of bacteria in my body, and my initial research led me to the book *The Yeast Connection* by Dr. William Crook. I learned that taking antibiotics causes the imbalance, and that sugar, yeast, fermented foods and starches feed the Candida yeast in the body. It was all starting to make sense. I was 26 years old and my diet consisted of beer, bread, Chinese food, tofu, and sugar in so many forms. I immediately removed all sugar, bread products, dairy, tofu, vinegar, soy sauce, mushrooms, potatoes, and beer from my diet. Most of my chronic symptoms went away, and I even lost ten pounds.

MORE THAN THE DIET

There were other items on the "avoid" list, such as birth control pills that I had been on since I was 16 years old. I ignored these, believing they really wouldn't matter. I also continued to drink liquor and wine after my month on the diet. I believed my Candida problem was under control because of the change in my diet. But a year later, a live blood analysis taken at a health food store indicated a lot of Candida in my body. I began a natural antifungal called Caprylic Acid and experienced enough positive reactions that I became fairly obsessed with Candida cleanses in a box.

During the following years, I continued to drink heavily, do drugs, and take birth control pills. At the same time, I loved juice fasting, colonics, and the world of wellness. I was also an over-achiever corporate sales chick filled with insecurity and low self-esteem, which I had tried to boost with breast implants at age 22. The most important thing to me was looking perfect because I thought it would make me lovable. My contradictory lifestyle took a toll on me. I became toxic, bloated, spacey, congested, and had frequent skin breakouts. Then I tried to remedy everything—including my shame—with a cleanse. This detox-retox cycle continued, and my bloating and brain fog worsened.

My relationship with men mirrored my dysfunctional relationship with myself. I ran off to Vegas to get married two weeks after I broke my engagement to another man. I knew I'd made a mistake after the first night of crazed fighting. I left the abusive marriage three months later and began wondering why I chose unhealthy relationships that robbed me of my power. To find out, I connected with my intuitive self during a weekend Inner Knowing Course. Over the next four years, I took every course they offered and eventually left my wildly successful corporate sales career (I was top three in the nation) to start my own business as a certified holistic health coach and journaling facilitator. Teaching journaling, health, and detox workshops in my living room created such clarity and bliss that I stopped my party girl life.

Still, something was not healing in my body. I was consistently bloated and constipated and having digestive problems and food sensitivities. I spent $5,000 for a week at a posh Ayurveda spa to purify my body and mind through panchakarma and was told to stop eating all raw foods. Two weeks later, I was more bloated than ever. I instinctively returned to only raw fruit and vegetables and became a raw foodist. I was eating the cleanest diet in the world and, again, feeling inspired and high on life. But with the frequent brain fog and craving for sugar, I knew I wasn't who I was supposed to

27

be. It was clear that I couldn't hold on to the life I had been living. I needed drastic change.

Through Julia Griffin's One True Self E-Course, I visualized myself on a tropical island doing what I love. After that, I sold everything I owned to leave my home in Atlanta and follow my heart to Thailand. I packed two pink suitcases and was guided to Koh Samui, an island that consisted of fourteen different detox retreats and thirty spiritual and energy healers. This was my paradise—filled with all my passions—on one beautiful tropical island. I decided to research all the retreats and healers and write a guidebook.

"YOU HAVE SYSTEMIC CANDIDA"

During my research, I experienced every practitioner on the island. An iridologist looked into my eyes and said the four words I had been waiting to hear my whole life: "You have systemic Candida." I knew it! I had been in some sort of denial until I was in the best situation to finally commit to whatever it took to heal. I was still eating a mostly raw food diet, so she told me to drink pau d'arco and avoid coffee, alcohol, and dried fruit. After a month, though, I didn't feel any different. I drank one glass of wine and got the flu.

At that point, my brain fog was at its worse. Since I knew the most about the detox retreats on the island, I was hired to create a wellness program for a resort that included self-awareness and spiritual healing. I was truly aligned and inspired, but I couldn't think clearly. That desire created my turning point. "I will do anything, whatever it takes, to think clearly," I told myself. The next day I was handed the *Body Ecology Diet* by Donna Gates. Donna explained how to rid the body of systemic fungal/yeast infection and how the healing process is different for everyone. It became my bible. The book also convinced me to eliminate alcohol completely.

Even though the island was full of detox and healing retreats, I was the only person on this type of diet. Nobody knew it like I did, even though I had just begun. The next month, I had no more strong cravings, my head felt clearer, and I had more energy. The diet created a new way of living for me—now I began to feel! I realized that I had gone my whole life numbing out on sugar, alcohol, drugs, sex, work, and shopping and being overly attached to "things." As repressed, uncomfortable emotions began to surface, I sought help from every healer on the island. I experienced Angel healings, hypnotherapy, spiritual releasing, and became attuned as a Reiki II practitioner. During one 10-day silent meditation retreat, I realized I needed long hair to be happy. Two weeks later, on New Year's Eve, I shaved my head. It was another step toward freedom.

GETTING RID OF THE VICTIM ENERGY

Through the combination of all of my work and healing, I started to notice negative patterns. Whenever I gave my power away to survive and created emotional stress with my thoughts, my bloating would get worse. I connected with Laura Bruno, a medical intuitive, who told me Candida resonates with "victim." She believed the key to my healing was to release any residual emotional and spiritual victim energy.

At the time, I didn't know what victim energy meant. Now I understand that whenever I felt stuck in a disempowered pattern with jobs or men or unhealthy behaviors, my Candida flared. Additional healing helped me deal with emotional pain and repressed anger, and soon I felt ready to leave Thailand. I followed the signs to San Francisco to work with the holistic community there.

DISCOVERING THE ROOT CAUSE

Living in San Francisco helped me continue my healing and research with the best spiritual, energy, and shamanic healers I could find. Then I left for a 30-day water fast in Costa Rica where I hoped to connect more deeply to my higher self and heart. During the fast, a man contacted me and asked if I would do a private detox program with him in Atlanta. I agreed. I came full circle back to Atlanta after three years, and after seven years of being single, I entered into what became another negative relationship that triggered the emotional root cause of my Candida: victimhood. I gave my power away to this man, lost trust in myself and in my business intuition, and settled for crumbs instead of the whole love pie.

Even though I was still eating a Candida-friendly diet, my bloating always worsened around him. He fed my victim condition. He was never emotionally available, and the hurt triggered me so deeply that yeast started to flow out of me. I realized at that point that the root of my Candida wasn't what I was eating; Candida was there because of what I *wasn't* feeling. Energy healer Janet Raftis confirmed that the deeper repressed negative emotions were holding that Candida in my body. The scared, insecure, unlovable girl inside me needed to feel safe and loved. Once I began acknowledging my inner child, loving her, and allowing her unresolved feelings–as well as the joy– to surface, all of my Candida symptoms and emotional eating soon went away. Now I could drink and eat what I wanted without any reactions. I no longer needed to be perfect or have the approval of others. I could just be me (and even had my breast implants removed). I also was ready to meet my soulmate, Doug Miller.

In retrospect, I was guided to Thailand, San Francisco, and Costa Rica so I could return to Atlanta to learn the physical, mental, emotional, and spiritual aspects of Candida and to fully heal and be empowered in every area of my life. Today I work with clients with chronic Candida and symptoms related to repression and disempowerment and who struggle, as I once did, with perfectionism, obsession with outside approval, unresolved trauma, and chronic victim mentality. But not everyone needs to address Candida on this level. Some have a Candida overgrowth simply because of antibiotic use, and can easily rebalance their gut with diet, antifungals, and probiotics.

If you are searching for your own healing, your body's wisdom and intuition are your biggest allies in the quest for the strongest you. Above all, be gentle with yourself. Release control of when you want your healing to happen and all expectations of how it's supposed to look. For once you believe you can heal yourself, the right resources will come to you. Have faith and pray.

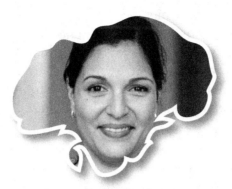

Anahi Brown

HHC, AADP, BSc

Anahi is a certified Wellness and Lifestyle Coach and Journalist with over 10 years of corporate experience working in radio, cinema and TV, in areas of writing, production and direction.

Currently, Anahi is working following her greatest passion, which is to support and empower women to regain their wellness, heal from within and thrive in life via her successful Wellness Coaching practice. Anahi is focused on enabling everyone around her to reach into their inner wisdom to discover what is it that they need to be happy, healthier and more joyful than ever before through her Holistic Nourishment approach, combining nutrition, emotional support, movement, quality rest and relationships work to obtain a full, rich and colorful life in the fast pace expat life in Qatar.

Her practice combines one on one coaching (both in person and through Skype), group coaching (special for people working through similar labels and beliefs), blogging, and her favorite: public speaking, both in diverse health and wellness themes as in cooking classes and demonstrations.

Anahi believes in achieving changes through a personalized transformative style that allows clients and followers to regain control of their wellness and joy so that they too can thrive in life using tools tailored for their own needs. In 2015, Anahi received the Ooredoo Sheroes award for her work supporting women going through Antenatal and Postnatal depression.

Contact Anahi:

www.anahibrown.com

🅂 **WellnessCoachAnahiBrown**

✉ **anahi@anahibrown.com**

🅕 **facebook.com/HealthCoachAnahiBrown**

🅣 **@anahi_brown**

📷 **@WellnessCoachAnahiBrown**

CHAPTER 4

HOW LOVE AND ACCEPTANCE INSPIRED MY HOLISTIC NOURISHMENT REVOLUTION

By Anahi Brown

As a little girl, I learned to speak very quickly. By 13 months, I was forming short sentences (mostly demanding my mother to nurse me in the middle of the night), and by two years, I could speak clearly, even correcting people who mispronounced my name. Apparently, I was not only fluent at speaking, I also LOVED it.

As the family stories go, I spoke all the time as long as I was awake. This funny fact won me the nickname Broken Radio. Funny, right? Not so much when you're a two year-old. I still remember the shame I felt whenever, in the middle of a conversation or round of questions, a relative would interrupt me to point out I spoke too much, that I was asking too many questions, that I was annoying. This is where my story starts.

You see, I come from a broken family with an abusive yet amazingly loving father and a powerful yet constantly terrified mother. No siblings, no pets. For my first six years of life, just the three of us and our drama. I have few happy memories of those years, yet plenty of bitter ones.

I remember seeing myself in the mirror, five years old, learning to read and write, seeing myself as flawed, as broken, as "insufficient," and sadly as fat. The funny thing is that when looking at pictures from back then, I see I wasn't, in fact I was perfect. Healthy, strong, tanned with rosy cheeks and shiny hair, and a sad gaze that still makes my husband feel sad of the "then-me" he never met.

By the time I was seven, my parents had separated; I was living with my mother under tough economic circumstances. I was steadily gaining weight, yet the most amazing part of my story, is the fact that by then I was beginning to diet. I was living with episodes of depression and social anxiety on a regular basis, especially when it came to interacting with my peers.

And so my life continued, I carried on gaining weight as well as experimenting with different weight-loss diets, loathing myself in all ways I could, feeling like an outcast, like a failure, yet excelling at school. One thing I always had going for me was that my marks were always great, as well as my sense of humor, as I assumed that as the "fatty" of the bunch, I had the obligation of being the funny one too (or as I like to call it the FFF—funny fat friend).

Among many things, I struggled with an eating disorder, depressive tendencies, and suicidal thoughts, which were particularly strong on my first years in college. While studying to be a journalist, I found myself surrounded by Miss Venezuela rejects who had the perfect and happy lives I never imagined I deserved due to my personality and weight.

I moved houses, cities, countries, and even continents, and finally, at 25 years, I found myself out of yet another abusive relationship. Depressed, lost emotionally and professionally, standing on the scale and realizing the months spent with an emotionally closed man who I felt rejected me, took its toll on my body and took me to my highest weight ever, almost 90 kg.

There I was, young but burdened by SO much, by my demons, by my self-hate, by economic problems that were beyond my control, fighting hard to continue fighting, even when all seemed lost. I had spent my life measuring my value on how much I weighed, if I had a boyfriend or not, how well I did in school or work, and how popular and loved I felt. Never realizing the fact that, as a young woman, I was amazing, powerful, kind, smart and unique, the fact that I was already perfect.

So, with my highest weight, my lowest self-esteem, and nothing to lose, I decided to go all-in: I was going to work my ass off to lose weight for real, to get healthy; I wasn't going to set a limit or push to lose 30 kg in two months like before, this time was all or nothing. I was going to learn to love exercise, eat better, and get healthier, regardless of what the scale said. I just wanted one last fight for my health.

I started exercising and counting calories. I also met Phil (funny how as soon as I said I was done dating for a while, this amazing Prince Charming showed up to change my mind), and we started dating. I was investing in myself for me, and at the same time, he started "loving me whole."

I'm convinced this was a turning point in my life; not only was I focused on living for myself only, working hard to be healthier, but also for the first time in my life, I had someone love me, approve of me, cherish me like never before, and that helped me heal… and so little by little, the weight started to come off.

It wasn't easy; it wasn't always fun either, but 18 months passed and I had lost 20 kg and couldn't believe it. Exercise was now a need, just as much as tracking every calorie I ate or "treating" myself to a nice dessert at the end of a good week.

I was engaged; I was in love; we had big plans and a wedding date, and I was thinner than ever, stronger, fitter, healthier but unhappy. Deeply unhappy. My days went between work, the gym, counting calories, and planning a wedding. Yes, I was no longer experiencing migraines as before, but still I felt I wasn't good enough, I wasn't thin or pretty enough.

So, there I was, on my wedding day, after overcoming countless step backs, about to promise my love and commitment to the man of my dreams, looking stunning and gorgeous, yet seeing the same fat girl that met me in the mirror over 20 years earlier, feeling I didn't do enough to be the perfect bride.

And I confess, that this same loathing continued for much of the first months of marriage. I had a near to perfect life, but felt disappointed at myself; I still didn't think I deserved this life. I was still lacking much… and then on January 5th, 2013, it happened. I suddenly had a positive pregnancy test. But, how could that be? I still needed to lose MORE weight; I still wasn't the person I wanted to be before becoming a mother, and I still felt broken.

During my pregnancy and for the first year of my son's life, I was intermittently depressed. When things were bad, I would spend weeks under the veil of sadness and loss. Then, suddenly I would have a good day, but soon enough I would crash again. After Matthew's birth, I also gained a lot of weight, and it felt like my health kept slipping out of my hands, regardless of what I did. I was studying to become a Health and Wellness Coach, yet I felt worthless, looked sick and fat, and could barely cope with motherhood.

It wasn't until Matthew was eight months that Phil lovingly confronted me with the fact that I had post-partum depression, and that I need help to overcome it. I began researching, started looking for information on how to nourish my body, how to recover from what felt like a living hell. In the following months I was also diagnosed with Hashimoto's Disease, an autoimmune form of hypothyroidism (basically my own immune system was attacking my thyroid every day). This label made SO much sense in my head, that I just married it, accepted it as part of who I was, as part of my essence and so I focused on how to be "less broken" with it, but never challenge it.

I got proactive, started working with a fantastic life coach, looked for a holistic practitioner who could support my body in healing, and started following groups, forums, and sites where I could learn more about depression, Hashimoto's, thyroid health, and motherhood. I was committed to heal, to make my life work and to recover, even though in the back of my mind, I thought I was too damaged to ever consider myself as normal.

Our diets changed, we went gluten, dairy, and sugar free. I also started taking many supplements to help my body recover (let's say that I took enough for my husband to say that I should have rattled when I walked). In fact the whole family was following different "healing protocols", even my son, I was on a mission to undo what I thought I had done wrong.

You might notice now that there was a lot of guilt in this process, a lot of wondering if I had made myself (and Matthew) sick. If my previous diets, the fact that I took oral contraceptives for 15 years, or that I used to take pills like candy had "broken" me, if it has also made Matthew less than perfect.

I saw both him and myself as patients, as walking diagnoses, as "damaged goods." Me with the Hashimoto's, the depression, the excessive talking, being overweight; him with his eczema, his low weight gain (ironic, I know!), his sleep issues, and the dark circles under his eyes. I focused on repairing what I felt was too messy; I set all my focus on disease.

Months went by and, although making steps forwards, I still lived with a lot of anxiety. Was I doing enough? Should I up my game? Did we need more supplements? Will we ever have a "normal" life again? The depression had subsided, but the weight didn't change much and my anxiety continued.

I used the diagnosis as an apology; I would speak at workshops about nourishment and health and say: "I'm overweight because I have a thyroid condition". It was the perfect excuse when I felt I wasn't doing enough to be thin and perfect, to be as I should have been.

One day, I started feeling tired. Very tired. I was trying to play with my then 19-month-old boy and could barely leave the bed. I had no energy, and panic filled my body, I immediately thought: "That's it, my thyroid is failing me, yet again." I remember speaking to Phil about it, telling him I was feeling really odd. I mean, I could have sworn I was pregnant, but the test came back negative, the doctor said that wouldn't happen easily due to my "condition," so it HAD to be my thyroid. I was really sick.

After all the deprivation from foods I used to enjoyed, after all the guilt, the work, the effort, here I was taking one step closer to losing control of my health thanks to my own body failing me, thanks to my immune system attacking the one part of my body it should have protected. I felt like a loser.

I started doubting the importance of all the commitments I had done, all that we did to keep Matthew and myself healthy, was that necessary? What was the point? I felt betrayed by my own biology… and so I hit back, with derailing from my "oh-so-perfect" diet, and once again doubting my body's ability to heal.

It took me a couple of weeks to return to sanity and re-shift my focus, and it all started with one (powerful) Reiki session. All of the sudden, I began to talk to like-minded people questioning what we knew of healing and diet, what we thought we understood about the role of nutrition in our conditions, in our health, and suddenly it made sense.

Even though, I worked convincing people of the importance of Holistic Nourishment in their wellness, the importance of stress and joy and how they can affect us more than whatever we eat, it had never really clicked in me until that day. And this wasn't because I had an amazing awakening or because God spoke to me, it was because I found myself holding another positive pregnancy test, against all odds, realizing how powerful and strong my body was, even when I refused to believe in it.

I had a new focus; my belief system had been shattered and was being rebuilt again, but now and for the first time in my life, I saw myself as whole, as powerful, as perfect, I saw my body as a perfect and powerful healing machine, where diagnoses were just labels that I could choose to let go of. I felt empowered in my own skin and that changed my life and our family forever.

My body, which months before felt like my own worst enemy, was finally acknowledged as my greatest ally. What I used to say to myself about my thyroid and its role on my reality changed, and now I would bless my thyroid, thanking it for everything it had done for me, for loving me, for keeping me going, for allowing me to place blame on it so that I could experience all these revelations and joys. I knew I was healthy, and suddenly, I started manifesting it.

Unexpectedly, the restrictions in our diets didn't feel like that, they felt like a conscious choice in supporting my ultimate health; the piles of supplements I took to "masquerade my body's inefficiencies" were also a choice; I didn't depend on them; they were like an extra I could take or let go, no more obsessing over them. Finally, what I thought was a place of failure and nothing but messes, turned into magic with the coming of our second child, my body was the holder of a new life, a new future, and that helped me realize its perfection.

All of this brings me here, to today, when we're expecting a new baby in December 2015, living with a new sense of power and wellness than shines from within, when I'm convinced all the labels have been stepping points in my road to understanding how powerful and perfect I have always been, when I focus on all of what's good and wonderful about myself and my family—physically, emotionally, mentally, and spiritually. Today, I know we are enough; we are strong; we are perfect; we are loved.

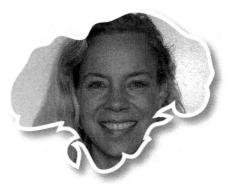

Janet Raftis

As an intuitive energy healer and coach, Janet Raftis helps her clients to navigate major life transitions through the process of releasing limiting patterns and beliefs from the past and shifting into a space of empowerment that allows them to realize their dreams. She works with clients from all over the world, and she has helped them move into new career paths, transition out of relationships that no longer serve them, develop their intuitive and spiritual gifts and more.

In addition to healing session work, Janet has developed individual and group programs that help women access their truth so that they may express it more fully in the world. She also holds meditation and women's circles and teaches spiritual development classes that provide others with the foundation to explore, open to their gifts and understand how those gifts can be of service to themselves and others.

Janet began healing work in 2004 as a way to heal from a rape and subsequent victimization and addiction issues. Her journey took her from feeling disempowered in most areas of her life to a space of gratitude and growth. She is a Reiki Master and has studied Pranic Healing and Matrix Energetics. As a psychic medium, she is able to see how past experiences have embedded themselves in her client's energetic field and to connect to each one's spirit team in order to receive individualized information to help them heal and grow. Janet's clients often refer to their work with her as expansive and life changing.

Janet has been published on elephant journal and the Manifest Station and maintains a blog on her website. She hosts a blog radio show on News for the Soul every second Tuesday of the month at 6:00 pm EST.

Contact Janet:

www.janetraftis.com

✉ **janet@janetraftis.com**

❶ **Janet Raftis—Healer and Author**

▣ **@JanetRaftis**

🐦 **@JanetRaftis**

CHAPTER 5

MAP TO HOME

By Janet Raftis

From a very young age, I felt responsible for everyone around me. I could feel what they were feeling, and I didn't know how to separate their emotions from mine, so I took responsibility for trying to change them. If I couldn't, I felt like I was to blame. I felt powerless, uncertain, and at-fault at every turn. Fear was my invisible companion; it went with me everywhere.

As fear and powerlessness followed me into adolescence, they began to pluck at me in a different way. They led me to drugs and alcohol and down paths that felt good in the moment but that always led to the same dead-end. I thought that I was liberating myself; the high carried me out of my body and into a state of perceived courage and aplomb. I felt invincible when I was intoxicated—strong and powerful, ready to take on the world.

And then I was raped. Afterwards, I slipped away. I stuffed my feelings, and I hid the event away in the recesses of my mind. I tried to move on, but in order to do so I actually shut down even more.

I stopped drinking for a long while after the rape. I dedicated myself to the tasks of studying and forgetting. But no matter how hard I tried, it didn't go away. I crawled into myself and disappeared in sweat pants and baggy shirts. I stopped wearing make-up, and I ceased to trust others. I finally moved across the country to escape a trail of wreckage that was causing me to feel personal torment and self-hatred.

I was looking for an escape, but I took my depressed and frightened self-right on to Atlanta, and within a few years, I was actively drinking and drugging again. I found myself once more in dysfunctional relationships and the after-effects of being raped were starting to leak out of me. I would cry during sex unless I was intoxicated. I was afraid to be in social situations, and I didn't trust anyone. My addictions escalated as I tried to shut myself down even more.

I met my (ex-) husband in the midst of this emotional climate, and after getting married, I tried another geographical change—my third at this point. We moved to Costa Rica, and after a year, I became pregnant. I took in the parallel pink lines at the end of the stick, and I dropped all of my vices—smoking, drinking, and drugs—from one second to the next, and I dedicated myself fully to the task of becoming a mother. I loved the experience of my son growing within me, but without the tools I'd been using to numb myself, a maelstrom of emotions rushed forth. I began to notice physical symptoms of disease. After my son's birth, my skin broke out and I was constantly bloated. Eating was becoming increasingly difficult because I felt sick after almost every meal. Within my marriage, I felt lonely, isolated, disempowered, and depressed.

I'd taken a peek at my rape every once in a while over the years, with the intention that maybe I would dig in a bit, but by the second or third glance, I'd quickly retreat back behind the cloak of denial. Finally, when my son was one, I began to study Reiki as a way to heal emotionally and physically. For the first time in my life, the pain was intense enough and the stakes were high enough that I actually gave it a sincere go.

As I did more energy work on myself and others, I began to notice connections between physical symptoms—I was suffering from a candida overgrowth—and emotions, though the full scope of the relation would remain a mystery for several more years. For the first time, I broached the anger and the fierce self-hatred that I had directed against myself while also doing the work to physically cleanse the excess yeast from my body.

During this time, I experienced a moment of clarity, and my husband and I separated after several years of being unhappy together. It was easy to think that now that my marriage was dissolving and I had cleansed myself physically, I would be healed. I wanted to believe that it could be that easy, but then there I was: the exact same reflection in the mirror stared back at me, and I still hated to look at it. I felt just as disempowered and weak as before, and all of my physical symptoms were returning.

I moved back to Atlanta, ripe with a vision for a new life that would magically unfold for me with minimal effort. I was going to pursue my vocation as a healer and travel the world helping to empower other women to heal themselves. Once back in Atlanta though my life began to unravel. I was still shut down and lost. I didn't know who I genuinely was, and I very quickly fell into prior patterns of behavior around addiction. I found work in a restaurant, I started to drink heavily again, I turned to men for validation of my worth through sex, and I completely shut myself off from the essence of me that had begun to peek out of her shell.

And then, about five months after my return, a miracle happened. During a late night fight with my ex (although separated, we were still very much in a co-dependent relationship), in which both of us were drunk and angry, our son woke up and called out for us to stop yelling. His father had been threatening to take him away from me. Ultimately, that threat was one of the greatest blessings of my life because at that moment a complete wave of surrender and grace washed over me. I felt it despite still being intoxicated. In that moment, the obsession to consume alcohol completely lifted. I felt profound peace and a sense of connection to Spirit that I hadn't known possible.

I found a support group the next day and began the work of living a sober life. I had gone through long periods of time in my life without drinking before, but my misery and fear had never lifted. Recovery provided me with a platform upon which I could actually begin to see myself clearly.

I began to love and appreciate myself for the first time, albeit in very small doses at first. I took baby steps, but at least I moved in the right direction. I began to notice more areas in my life where I was disempowered as I once more began to experience the physical symptoms of bloat and exhaustion.

Again, I reached a critical point with my health. I could barely function, and I felt overwhelmed by the simplest tasks. Even getting up off the couch seemed difficult at times. In desperation, I scoured the Internet looking for a solution, and I was led to a Nutritional Response Therapist. My sense of fear and disempowerment had always left me heavy with financial fear so investing in my health was a huge step for me. My NRT specialist uncovered a variety of food, chemical, and environmental sensitivities that were compromising my system along with a recurrence of candida.

I underwent the physical healing through dietary changes and supplements, and I fully engaged in the work to heal the underlying emotional causes of my illnesses and –isms. I ripped apart my fears and started to systematically move through them.

I felt better than I had in years. This was a key piece for me and one that I was able to explore more fully through work I did with Elicia Miller: candida and digestive disorders are physical manifestations of disempowerment. Being raped by guys I had thought were friends in a situation I had deemed safe followed by two other near rapes in the ensuing years had left me in a state of complete disempowerment. I had no trust in myself, and I felt like life happened to me instead of through me.

I had believed that others had more control over me than I did and that I was helpless. I couldn't speak up and I lived in constant fear that there wouldn't be enough money, love, friendship, *anything*. I had a hard time expressing my true authentic self because I had no idea who I was. A lifetime of fear had taught me to hide, to become invisible, to bleed into the background.

To overcome the fear, I vowed to do one thing every day that scared me. This flexed my faith muscle and I began to feel courageous and strong. I actually started to put myself out into the world in a new way. I continued my personal healing, and I attacked my patterns, limiting beliefs, and behaviors with fervor. I vowed that I would never live in that darkness again—a promise that is still a motivating factor for me as I move through my life.

The empowerment aspect was the piece that had eluded me for all those years, and it is what had affected me on emotional, physical, mental, and spiritual levels. My life is rich now. I have deeper and more fulfilling relationships. I adore the work I'm doing. My finances are healthier than they have ever been. I love my home and my neighborhood. When I look around me, I feel good. When I look in the mirror, I feel love. And I realize that everything that is outside of me looks and feels great because the inside of me feels better than ever.

My healing is not done, but it has opened up enough that I am able to explore myself with curiosity and love and that, to me, is the absolute best place to be. Finally, I am at home in me.

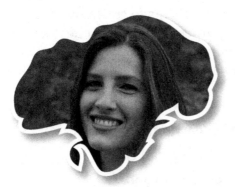

Jessica Al Andary, IAHC

Jessica is a Holistic Health Coach who empowers women who have been injured by life to step back into their Resilience, ignite their Healing and create a life of Joy.

At 24 she survived a car crash that left her with brain injury and a pelvis fractured in four places. Having to redesign her life in every way, she embraced a life-long passion for healthy eating and graduated from the Institute of Integrative Nutrition with a certificate in Health Coaching.

Today she lives with chronic pain though she chooses to think of it as *just another challenge* and aspires to create abundance in her life despite it.

Focusing on each meal as a vital element to healing—creating the best environment on a cellular level to allow your body to heal—is a core belief. She strengthens her body through Movement and Mindful Practice. Investing in her Support Network of friends, Mentors and Coaches allows her to grow her own business whilst caring for her husband and active young son.

Jessica supports her clients to create rituals that serve their ultimate meaning and purpose in life despite their personal challenges. Through her programs and workshops she offers personalized plans, accountability and understanding to create a life of Bliss.

Contact Jessica:

www.JessicaAlAndary.com

✉ **jessica.alandary@gmail.com**

ⓕ **facebook.com/jessica.andary**

CHAPTER 6

A CHANGE FORCED UPON ME

Jessica Al Andary

"Ok!" I think, "I'll do better next time." I'm always pushing the boundaries to see if I am stronger. It's so hard wanting to achieve goals and just not physically being able to. I have discipline, well except for when it comes to chocolate. I have knowledge, passion, ambition, inner joy. Today, I am being patient, still loving my broken body. Trying not to think of myself this way.

Life is not always like this. These days, for months at a time, I feel great rather than injured. I have learnt how to work with my body to live an amazing life; to manage my expectations and be realistic about my capabilities.

But right now in the depths of pain, all I have is my breath and staying calm; the knowledge that this moment too will pass.

I have learned to listen to the warning signals, to acknowledge my body's call for rest. Sometimes I think I can overcome my challenges by sheer willpower, but then my body reminds me the process is simple: Eat vibrant, life-giving foods, move often, and rest.

There was a time when I had my whole life ahead of me, my own imagination the only obstacle. It all changed in a fraction of a second. On a Friday night, exactly one week into my two week vacation in South Africa and one day before one of my closest friend's wedding, my fiancé and I were driving over 1000 km from my parent's home in the Eastern Cape to Cape Town—a city filled with vibrant life. I was excited to share this city with Wassim. We were working in the Kingdom of Saudi Arabia, and even though it was a luxurious resort owned by the Royal family, it was no match to the beauty of Cape Town.

My life was exciting and right on track: I had recently started working as a Restaurant Manager abroad–my dream of working and exploring the world had begun. Even more recently, I had gotten engaged to a special man and felt my friend's wedding was a perfect opportunity to introduce him to my family and the country of my heart, South Africa.

We had chosen to drive to Cape Town to see more of our naturally diverse country and to jump off the world's highest free-standing bungee jump. At 216 meters high, it was quite the scariest and most exhilarating thing I had ever done.

My memory of the day goes thus far. As we saw the lights of Cape Town and were so close to the Guest House with the Sea View Room, I have only the memories Wassim has shared with me. In that time, another driver sped through a red light and crashed into us, knocking us both unconscious.

Wassim woke to someone ripping his bracelet off. At first what he thought was people trying to help, turned out to be people robbing us! Helpless, perhaps dead, these poor people thought to take what they could rather than try to save our lives.

Between my fiancé trying to understand what had just happened, trying to get out of his seat, and trying to stop the people "shopping in our car," he was also trying to wake me and I was not responding. His instinct, refined by working in Fire and Rescue for years, kicked in.

Moments passed, then another driver stopped to help, a tow truck driver alerted the authorities, and the police and an ambulance arrived.

Wassim called my parents, the only people he knew in the country. The only words my mother heard from him were, "We were in an accident. Jessi's ok, Jessi's ok," and then the phone cut—the battery was flat.

But I was not ok.

My parents sat helplessly so far away, the worst fear of any parent: your child is hurt and you know not where or how and can do nothing about it. They waited until, finally, at 3 am the hospital called and told them I was severely injured: I was in a coma; there was bleeding on the brain, and there was no way to predict if I would live or die.

That was 9 years ago, and I survived.

The next year was one filled with intense recovery, love, and support. I was mentally knocked down a few times, of course, especially when a specialist told me one leg would be shorter than the other (which wasn't true) and that I may never be able to carry a child.

My parents were further distressed as I did not have medical insurance; my insurance in Saudi Arabia didn't cover me in South Africa, and I hadn't thought to take travel insurance. My fiancé, family, friends, and acquaintances donated, and our town even had a golf day to raise funds for my hospital bills and continued medical expenses. My mom took three months off work to care for me.

Even though I didn't have a visible scratch on me, the head injury was severe. Once I survived the four day coma, I developed short term memory loss, along with double vision. When doctors could focus on more than just my head injuries, they discovered four fractures in my pelvis. Nothing could be done to repair it, so I had 6 weeks of bed-rest, and we just had to wait and see. I had to lie flat-on-my-back for six weeks—think nappies, bedpans, muscle loss, and complete dependence.

The short term memory loss was scary for my family—was it permanent?! In the beginning I would forget things I had been told just moments before. My first post-accident memory is from two weeks after the accident. My parents were around me in the bedroom, and I asked them to leave the room as I needed to relieve myself. When they were outside, I decided to go to the toilet—I had forgotten I couldn't walk and when I tried to get out of bed, I fell flat on my face. A plastic surgeon happened to be nearby and (mostly) straightened my broken nose.

A year after the accident, the orthopedic surgeon told me simply: Due to the force of the crash directly on my side, my pelvis is now skewed and not all the bones re-connected. I will always have pain; it is up to me how I choose to live my life.

Learning at 23 that I will have to endure a lifetime of pain was a scary, debilitating realization. I had always been active, participating in sport and outdoor activities. And as tough as the prognosis was to understand and process, the doctor's words have also been empowering when I looked at it in a different way.

His words have allowed me to get up again and again when I fell to the depths and to realize I am not doomed to a life of suffering. I have a choice—perhaps not the kind I had before, but I still have control over my life. If something doesn't work, I explore the reason and learn how to do things differently. Often the answer was to increase my boundaries, to learn to say "no" when I need to (not that I necessarily want to). Having a circle of support and love has allowed me to hold onto my dreams and tap into my inner strength when times get tough. One of my mentors is my dad, Ivan, who was paralyzed at 21. A parabat in the army at the time, he had been rock-climbing the day he had a motorbike accident. Despite his immense disability, he has traveled, explored, and LIVED; he has been a source of strength, empathy, and inspiration.

Since I was young, I was interested in healthy eating. Interestingly for me, the year I was recovering I just wanted to eat life-giving foods, even more than before. I wasn't even interested in chocolate which had been my life-long craving. I just wanted soup and fruit and salad. I lost some extra weight I had been carrying since I was 18—a little consolation prize perhaps.

Wassim and I got married in Cyprus 11 months after the accident, and we moved to Islamabad, Pakistan. A new adventure! I was now ready to get back to life as a Restaurant Manager at the Marriott Hotel. My parents thought it was a mistake going back to work so soon, and in some ways, they were right. Physically, I couldn't manage; I shed many tears coming to terms with my new body and so much pain. My husband was (still is) so supportive; he was THERE when everything changed and understood (perhaps better than me). For the next 3 years, we changed countries and jobs three times; Wassim would try anything to help me.

The hospitality industry with its long, demanding hours was not sustainable, and eventually, the reality of my injuries set in. I could not live the same life as the one I had planned. I hated the idea of "chronic pain" and tried as many different therapies and healing modalities as I could find: Physiotherapy, Chiropractor, Osteopathy, Homeopathy, Allopathic medicine, Crano-sacrul therapy, Hydrotherapy, Acupuncture, Aromatherapy, Healing massage, Myofacial triggerpoint therapy, Dry Needling. Medicine hasn't really helped, so I have had to explore deeper ways of healing. All of these therapies have helped me in different ways over the years. As we moved many times, the first thing I do when we are settled in a new place is to find a therapist with whom I resonate. Mostly the "standard" physiotherapy available through insurance was not enough for my body, so I found therapists who would treat me in private practice. The cost was worth it; because to feel good in my body, strong and supple, allows me to face the world again with a smile. Part of my self-care now is to go for a massage and alignment (osteopath or chiropractor) every month and though it is expensive, it has given me quality of life back.

Since the doctor gave his first ok, I started doing physical therapy flat on my back to assist the healing process. Movement and strengthening are important tools I use—swimming, walking, personal training, Pilates, Yoga. A "Yoga for Emotional Balance" course taught me to trust my body and the power of my breath. Mindfulness has allowed me to access my own resilience—in the times when pain is severe, when I didn't listen to the warning signals, my breath, patience, and self-love through gratitude practice are healers.

We spent five years in Qatar, and this is where I was able to create a life of meaning and purpose again. I met a like-minded soul who has been instrumental in me finding my self-confidence. Nicole is amazing—energetic, passionate about Holistic Health and wanting to heal the world—she was (is) a real catalyst for change. Our paths crossed at the right time, she introduced me to the concept of Holistic Health and through her support and friendship I decided to study through the Institute of Integrative Nutrition, the largest nutrition school in the world, and learnt that healthy eating is so much more than the food you put in your mouth.

My journey has been a tough one. I have realized no one has it "easy," everyone has their own struggles and deserve empathy. I reached a point a few years ago when I decided I am not going to let my injuries define me any longer. I will live a productive, joy-filled life. I have learnt to be patient with myself. I can perhaps not work as many hours as other people can, but I still have value to give the world. Turning 30 was an amazing year in my life: I graduated from the Institute of Integrative Nutrition as a Holistic Health Coach, and I gave birth to a healthy, happy boy!

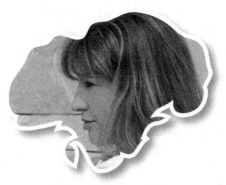

Emily Alp

Emily is a science writer by trade, and a Yogini, health researcher and expressive, altruistic person by nature. Through her 12-year journey to discover celiac disease at the root of her health challenges, she explored a range of literature and approaches to human health and wellbeing. The discovery of celiac was only the beginning of claiming and rebuilding her health, and momentum in this direction—discovering ways to maintain personal balance and enhance quality of life on all levels—has proven to be a life calling. She continuously discovers new health secrets and shares these as well as anything in life she finds beautiful, inspiring or positively moving. She believes health is also a matter of attitude and that flexibility on all levels, a desire to find meaning in all situations, and a willingness to embrace change and life as a learning process are essential keys to maintaining it. As a recent step in her training to become a holistic life coach, she signed up for year-long program to become a nutrition adviser. Currently, she is a Yoga instructor with specializations in Ayurveda and Pranayama. Considered Yoga's sister science, Ayurveda is a several thousand year-old, highly-practical system that offers a fresh perspective on the human system as a whole. Pranayama is a way to address the body through controlling the breath, which is intimately linked to the nervous system. These studies have enriched not only her Yoga practice but also her life overall. She continues to study and teach asana-based and breath-based classes in Doha, Qatar, and freelances to share new insights with the public.

Contact Emily:

www.Emilyalp.com

f **facebook.com/emily.alp**

@emilyalp

@emilyalp

CHAPTER 7

TO KNOW THE LOST SEASHORE

By Emily Alp

When I see baby sea turtles push up out of the sand and watch their flippers pinwheel frantically, I feel deep resonance. I know what they're after. I connect with that sheer will to live. I know what it is like to try to make it to the sea in modern times.

Once upon a hundred years ago, the sky was filled with only stars and moonlight to cue the tiny turtle's instincts; now streetlights and shop fronts shine loud, confusing its natural, intuitive, age-old navigation system. Likewise, we humans can only imagine a time before foods became so processed we needed five minutes to read their labels, often finding ourselves sicker for eating them. A time before doctors were paid by pharmaceuticals to push drug-based distractions from solutions that could lead us to the sea of our lives. I know what it's like. And so do many of you.

Like the sea turtles, I also know what it's like to part with a mother early. Fortunately, life's ocean offered circumstances and caregivers to nurture, support, and urge me early to understand: there comes a time to shake off your parents and the past as influences that might distract your willpower when navigating to the waters of your life and future.

I was a naïvely open and deeply sensitive child. Mom left us with dad when I was about two. My bond with her—well remembered to this day—was otherworldly. To me, she was an archetypal goddess. My lungs shut down from grief within days after she left. She visited and snuggled me in the oxygen tent at the hospital before saying goodbye again—something I have come to understand was as difficult for her as it was for me.[1]

Meanwhile, deep within my cells, my genes wove a mysterious GI condition called celiac, which, by its complex autoimmune twists and turns, was fueled by eating wheat … and compounded by stress. The more stress, the more swatches of my small intestines would get inflamed, leaky, and retarded in terms of their ability to absorb nutrients.[2] The roots of this mysterious condition would elude me for years, however.

Symptoms began in childhood, masquerading as a deficient immune system—asthma managed by a couple of inhalers and some emergency room ventilation pipe sessions, as well as severe allergies. Pictures of me until about age 15 feature spindly arms and legs and a bit of an anemic complexion. I was able to eat more than boys my age and yet not gain a pound. Stomach cramps, bloating, bouts of pain and fainting (usually after a big bowl of wheat cereal) marked these years, but I was a very fired-up girl and was too busy running around, playing, and exploring to dwell on it.

In high school, I loved martial arts, the 200 in track and field, and volleyball. These were ventilation outlets for the heat of teenage angst. And they worked. Socially, I was docile. I was living with my aunt and her family, provided for and engaging in sports that boosted my confidence—what did I know yet about the real stresses of making a living?

Then came the ultimate competition—with my own devices, at university. I got into nursing school, something I thought I "should" do. The science, math, and anatomy courses demanded everything from me, and I craved excellence. Stress, lost sleep, less exercise, binge beer drinking, and pizza threw me into so much intestinal pain that I could barely sit still in lectures. Still, I was on the dean's list and heading toward a prestigious internship.

I began to lose weight due to a general sense of apathy toward eating anything. As I did, I latched onto deprivation as a control mechanism. Enter, in hindsight, what I would say was more than a brush with anorexia. I maintained an "I'm just fine" disposition while my size plummeted from a US five to a zero within about eight months. My grades sored through the roof, however. "Everything is perfectly under control," said my imagination.

Concerned, my aunt took me to the doctor. He took five minutes to conclude that I should avoid fats and then prescribed muscle relaxants (which I took for a day and then threw away). In the summer after my freshman year, my cousin was in the bathroom with me when I slipped the clothes off my size zero frame and stepped into the shower. Horrified by my personal concentration camp cameo, she got the family together. An intervention ensued.

They sat quietly, carefully, in a circle around me: Was I happy at school, with my life, with what I was doing? These questions, which I never granted myself the right to ask, flooded me with a sense of relief as the answers raced out of my mouth: I wasn't at all passionate about becoming a nurse. Why was I doing this to myself then, they asked.

Relieved, I dropped out of school, and my aunt signed me up for an eating disorder program, wherein I was weighed regularly and taught to keep a food diary based on portions and food groups vs. relentless calorie counting. I will never forget filling out depression and eating disorder survey with the question: "Do you wipe off your chewing gum to cut calories?" In that moment I felt awestruck by the precision of this disorder that I was a confirmed member of.

I eagerly attended cognitive therapy sessions with an unforgettable woman, Nancy, who tapped me into the workings of my mind, the possible other realities besides the ones I latched onto, and my ability to ask myself questions instead of subsist on narrow assumptions. Every session with her, I grew more fond of our talks, until about two months in, when she shut her notebook at the end of a discussion, looked up at me and said—"Emily, you are smart enough to have these conversations with yourself. I foresee one, maybe two minor relapses, but you will get through, and you will make it."

MY LIFE—A.K.A. MY RESEARCH PROJECT

I never saw Nancy again, but her words echoed as an explanation for two future bouts of anorexic-grade control of my diet. As she predicted, the bouts were shorter, and I dug myself out swiftly. In addition to researching the root cause of the stomach problems, I was struggling to develop some kind of working relationship with something I couldn't survive without, yet was the source of immense abdominal pain: food.

Meanwhile, I had student loan debt and no real direction, so I spent five years waitressing, bartending, and learning how to drive my life. It was at this time that I was able to devour anything written about health and nutrition. Amidst herbal bibles and books on a range of diets, I found myself listening to the audiobook of *When Food is Love*, by Geneen Roth. Open, desperate, I followed her example for a year: eating anything I wanted, whenever and however much I wanted, gaining whatever weight came, and accepting myself without linking diet to appearance.

It was worth it, and after that year, I felt it was great but that I was heavy and had enough radical diet freedom. I was ready to structure my eating and life again. I created an exercise routine and chose foods that were enjoyable and easy to digest; foods that gave me energy and helped me feel light vs. dogmatic, diet-fad, one-approach-fits-all hearsay. As a massive bonus, I began to tear down the life-or-death need for other people's approval about my appearance.

But I was still in pain—so much so that my life still felt more like an experiment than actually doing what other people took for granted: simply getting up in the morning and living. My social life was only hinting at this. I didn't tell anyone about the pain as it was embarrassing to talk about. I was just the hippy girl at work who spent the extra money at Whole Foods, didn't eat meat, and didn't drink soda. I also picked up a pair of running shoes and joined a fellow bartender to try a half marathon. It was easy for me, so I trained for a full marathon and ran three of them in the course of a year and a half. Professionally, I had worked my way up to high-end wine bars, so the waitressing and bartending profession became a thick glass ceiling. I sensed my own potential and needed more out of life.

Feeling tested, tired of pain, and deeply exhausted, I was teetering on depression. While eating an egg one morning, one of my molars fell out, and I knew that my body was unable to get the minerals it needed despite the care I took to feed it. I recall at this time walking into a new age bookstore I loved. I had little money, but I decided to purchase a Yoga book. Many people can say that a teacher turned them on to Yoga, but for me it was a pose: I recall enjoying most the boat pose, in Sanskrit "Navasana." Today—over a thousand teacher-trainer hours later—I smile deep inside every time it graces my life. I owe so much to that beautiful, unassuming pose. Truly, it mesmerized me with its new level of mind-body sophistication. And thus began a gradual turn in the road toward an intuitive relationship with my body that I desperately craved.

I decided to go back to University around then, and it was at this time, fortunately, that I discovered an acupuncturist named Dr. Zhou, from China. His needlework focused on the spleen point on the inside of my leg just below the knee, as well as direct stomach points. I wasn't sure what would happen, but I found it relaxing, and I had to stay open minded as I continued my research to crack my life's code. After all, what other options were there? Muscle relaxants? The removal of my intestines?!

Then in one visit to Dr. Zhou, my whole life changed. I'll never forget it. He was holding my wrist, taking my pulse, and he asked me to stick out my tongue. He looked at it and looked at me and said, nonchalantly: "Emily, you stop eating bread rolls; start eating sweet potato." In that moment, I experienced what I love to call "superbrain." My thoughts raced with his insights to memory of something I read in a single paragraph of the regularly updated and ever-in-print tome *Prescription for Nutritional Healing*. After all this, could it be, WHEAT?!

FREEDOM

Full of hope, I started another elimination diet, hunting down information on what foods—and food additives—contained wheat. Like a computer programmer, I locked these into my mind and shopped slower, reading every label. I knew it would take time for such an experiment to show results, so I stuck to it. About a month into this elimination diet, I felt something wild happening. The pain that had hallmarked most of my life to that point was gone, for a day or two and soon a week, and soon longer. And when it showed up, it was not the same. It wasn't so distracting or demanding or exhausting.

My emotions were mixed. I realized I was finally saying goodbye to a huge part of my life, i.e., consuming levels of pain and the mission to find its source. Luckily, I could sink into challenging courses at school and had also started Yoga classes. I felt a love for Yoga forming in the background of academic work and internships. Over the years, this love grew into a passion as I moved first to New York City and then abroad as a science writer Yogini.

These days, most of my vacations—from work as a science book editor—involve Yoga trainings, Ayurveda courses, and detoxes in India and Thailand. Every day, I spend time meditating on gratitude, and most days I dedicate a couple hours to deepening my breathing, my concentration, and my relationship with my body through passed-down practices. I find these Yogic practices, when one is dedicated, work very gradually to promote integrity within, to align body, mind, and soul. These activities satisfy me, because for some reason I was born into a life demanding faith, will, and intuitive reasoning. Since my time with Dr. Zhou, I have opened myself to many healers—acupuncturists, chiropractors, bio-energy workers, Ayurvedic doctors, intuitive shamans, and friends. I still experience milestones in the rebuilding of my health and the integration of what I learn in all areas of my life—socially, emotionally, intellectually, physically, spiritually. All are connected, all reveal themselves in perfect time for me to live a little more—and to realize every morning, as I hatch open a new day, I have only just begun.

NOTES

[1] My relationship with my parents went through a similar transformation, in parallel with my physical, mental, and emotional health breakthroughs. I would not trade a moment of my life or any member of my family with anyone else's.

[2] Great read: Fasano, A. (2009). Celiac Disease Insights: Clues to Solving Autoimmunity. Study of a potentially fatal food-triggered disease has uncovered a process that may contribute to many autoimmune disorders. *Scientific American Magazine*, July 27.

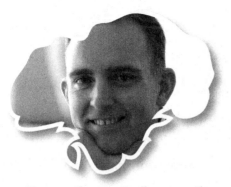

Jacob Melaard

For over five years, Jacob has helped hundreds of people achieve unprecedented levels of health and happiness. Known for his warm smile, caring demeanor and his ability to forge safe spaces where people can share, grow and feel free, Jacob loves nothing more than getting to know people and then triggering reactions that bring out the very best. He is a passionate, results-driven coach who is also known as a trusted partner among those seeking the power to gain confidence, lose weight, reduce stress and to find more fulfillment from this thing we call the human experience. Jacob's highly-acclaimed workshops and retreats have become celebrated for their ability to reshape the way people think about themselves, their careers, and how they can make a difference in the world around them.

Jacob is an NLP master practitioner, master hypnotist, and certified Strategic Intervention Coach via the legendary Anthony Robbins coaching school. He is an expert in blending cutting-edge techniques from the fields of neuro linguistic programming, Time Line Therapy, hypnosis and psychology. He is also a level 2 practitioner in emotional freedom techniques. He has been the wellness coordinator for Six Senses spa in Doha for over 3 years and prior to launching his career as an acclaimed transformational coach, Jacob spent 18 years serving as a renowned head chef in five-star hotels around the world.

When he isn't spending time with clients, Jacob enjoys golf, cooking and spending time with his family.

Contact Jacob

www.jacobmelaard.com

www.dropweightfeelgreat.com

⑤ jacob.melaard

✉ jacob@jacobmelaard.com

f facebook.com/jacob.melaard

in linkedin.com/pub/jacob-melaard/1b/330/922

CHAPTER 8

I WILL DO IT!

By Jacob Melaard

"Try and sit on the chair," he said it for the seventh time and I was feeling anxious, scared, confused, and just wanted to sink into the ground and never come back up. The 30 other people in the room giggled and laughed at my discomfort and I said in desperation, "Tell me what you want me to do. I DON'T GET IT!"

On a quiet February night in 1999, I was at an information evening about emotional balance, a combination of therapies and techniques that works on "everything". To demonstrate the process, the facilitator asked for a volunteer to show the processes, and I enthusiastically raised my hand. I wanted to stop smoking and had tried many times before but just couldn't kick the habit. This was going be a quick fix! Or so I thought.

Ten minutes later, I was in the center of a stage and the practitioner was asking me to say things like "I love and accept myself", tapping with his fingers on my face and ears, and asking me through muscle testing if it was something in my childhood that caused me to smoke.

I was hot, I was cold, I was emotional, and I was glad it was over. I also really wanted to light up a cigarette.

His question to me was simple,

"Are you going to stop smoking?" And my reply was equally simplistic, "I will try."

He then placed a chair in the center of the stage and told me to "try and sit on the chair." Me, being a person who likes to please and do what I am told, complied and quickly sat down.

"No, no, no, get back up, and try to sit on the chair" Said the man who, besides being an emotional balance expert obviously was also a comedian.

And again, I sat down and was asked to get back up and try to sit down.

I didn't get it. "What does he want me to do?" and "I didn't sign up for this," were some of the thoughts going through my mind. So after seven times of this game I said, "Tell me what you want me to do. I DON'T GET IT!"

He then explained that me saying "I will try" equals "I'm not going to do it" as we cannot "try" anything. We do, or we do not (I later realized that a famous character in the movie Star Wars said these exact words to save the galaxy from the dark side, so it must be true).

It was the metaphorical penny that dropped.

"I DO IT!!! I will stop smoking now!" I told him and all the people in the room. I walked out, leaving my cigarettes behind, and I've never looked back and never smoked again since. This was in 1999.

It was a moment of complete transformation. One I would be recreating many times over in the future with my clients. However, at that time, I was "happily" cooking professionally and living in my small hometown. Shortly after this transformational experience, I moved from my small rural village in the country side of Holland, to Florida in the U.S.A.

It was as if I got a second chance at life (and I was only 25). A whole new world of opportunities and possibilities opened up for me. I met new people, spoke a new language, worked in a new location, and I even had time to enjoy all there is to enjoy in Florida. From beaches to theme parks, and Michelin star food to junk-fast food.

Also detaching myself from "home" and the comfort zone that I got accustomed to all these years was making me feel that this could be a new beginning for me.

I had a passion for travel, for new experiences, and, I thought, for being a chef. Note the word "thought."

Growing up, I never knew what I wanted to be, so I always just did whatever would please others. During my time in vocational education, I didn't know what I wanted. I only knew what I didn't want. That was obvious. I didn't want to be lonely and alone. So after the first two years in vocational college where I was exposed to all kinds of professions (working with wood, metal, cooking, electronics, etc.), I chose electronics. Not because I wanted to, but because it was what my friends were choosing.

Needless to say, I had a tough time learning and understanding electronics as they didn't excite me one bit. I graduated from my class and then decided to become a chef.

My brother, who is 18 months older than me, is a chef. He is very different from me, and I always had the feeling that he got more attention than me. (This was not the case, but this was how I experienced it.) In order to please and get love, I decided to become a chef just like him. Obviously, this didn't change a thing in my experience of feeling loved. It just made me feel more uncomfortable.

Because I wanted to keep up and get the recognition and love I wanted and needed from my parents (and no, there is no judgement here...), I became a chef.

My passion for cooking, however, was nothing more than a way of serving, helping, and pleasing people–My staff, my bosses, the guests who ate my food. I rose to the top of my profession. Leading and managing kitchens with over 25 chefs. All in 5 stars resorts in top class locations in the Caribbean, Spain, Dubai, and London. I was known as "the calm one." I like to think I was a kind and caring person, who was generous with his time to his staff and his peers.

Because of the "stop smoking experience" in '99, I invested years of study into learning how the brain works. How is it that we can change in an instant? Why do some of us change and others don't? I learned about Reiki, psychology, meditation, mindfulness, and many other self-help techniques. I did all this so I could help my team more effectively.

In 2010, I reached the proverbial fork in the road.

I was in a job that I didn't like, because I was doing it for the wrong reasons and was 15 kilos overweight. Despite all the learning, I didn't feel good. I had anxiety over my job, and not enough time with my young family. My son was born in 2005, and I was away a lot of time. When you work in professional kitchens, most of the time you work when everyone else is having time off. Bottom line, I was unhappy, even though for the outside world it seemed as if I had it made.

Was this what I wanted to teach my son?

Was I going to create memories with him?

Would I live to see him grow up if I continued this lifestyle?

I realized that if I continued to destroy myself by ignoring what it is that I really want for me, if I keep looking after everybody but myself, I will not live the life I want or leave the legacy I want.

At the end of a course in Neuro Linguistic Programming (NLP), I made the decision to quit my job.

That job had given me so much in terms of seeing the world and doing extraordinary things in extraordinary places, but it filled me with anxiety, fear, and pain.

It was time to start helping people as a transformational coach.

I moved to Spain and studied Emotional Freedom Technique (EFT), also known as tapping, and within 6 months, I lost over 17 kilos (38 lbs) of body weight.

The most remarkable part was that it happened without any change in diet or lifestyle. In fact, I started to eat more by having regular meals, instead of no food for a full day and eating just at dinner time.

I realized again, it is the beliefs we hold and the thoughts we think that create our level of wellness. Of course, diet and exercise play a part, but my estimate is that 80% of weight control is mind-set, the other 20% is food and exercise. I started using my powerful brain to help me on my path to health and wellness.

The struggle with weight, is that most people can release (or lose) it, but cannot keep it off, unless they eat only lettuce and steamed onions, or whatever the fad diet is that people buy into.

I discovered that it is about the way we live our lives and the way we use or brains that makes us either release or gain weight.

It is my personal and professional experience that permanent and long lasting physical and psychological wellness starts when we get happy and fulfilled by releasing our negative beliefs and emotions.

It starts by committing to yourself. It starts when you say and believe "I WILL DO IT"!

CHAPTER 9

THEY CALL IT BLOOD SUGAR, SO WHY ISN'T THIS SO SWEET?

By Mario Ballesteros

What? AGAIN??

This has to be the fourth bathroom stop on the trip. What the HELL is this all about? Combined with an insatiable appetite, I was still losing weight. You'd think dropping those excess pounds would make me feel better. But I was feeling worse and worse.

I soon found out what it was all about. A visit to the doctor and a blood test said it all…..Type II Diabetes. I jokingly said, "Looks like Dad's disease finally caught up with me." But this was no joke. My sugar readings were an off-the-chart 500 (normal is 100), and the doctor told me to get on insulin and oral medication immediately. Somehow I knew my life was going to change and not for the better.

I stomped around for a week or so about not being able to eat the things I wanted all the time. And then my wife Linda got very hard with me and said if I did not want to be like my father I had to make some hard dietary changes, immediately. I wish I could say I got on board right away but I cannot. There was a little pushback on my side. All right I gave Linda a LOT of pushback, I am sorry to say. Looking back, I feel kind of embarrassed at my actions. After all I did not smoke, drink, or take drugs. My "drug of choice" was food. Texas barbecue, the Tex-Mex cuisine I grew up on, and oh yes, I was an incredible ice cream hound. I didn't take kindly to hearing that these all had to go away and this was going to be my life for the foreseeable future.

But then I thought long and hard about my Dad's last year of life, especially his last months. Long ignored side effects of his diabetes had ravaged his body. His legs ached all the time from the neuropathy which eventually left him unable to walk. He was in constant pain. Even worse, his kidney functions had quit, and he suffered the indignity of having to wear adult "garments" that made him feel like a helpless baby. For a proud Mexican gentleman, this was awful to see. They say no one actually dies from diabetes; it's the complications that kill you. Oh joy.

But I saw this was about to become ME if I did not take drastic steps. So I slowly started cutting back on my starches and sweets, grumbling all the while. This wasn't coming easy, at least at first. I had started my oral medications plus the nightly insulin shots. And did I mention the several times a day blood sugar readings? Damn that hurt until I learned how to do it right! You'd think that would "incentivize" me. Between the test strips and meter for blood sugar readings, the orals meds, the insulin injector and needles my side of the bathroom looked like a pharmacy. Not a pretty sight for someone who previously never took anything more than the occasional aspirin.

Progress was very slow. My blood sugar readings were still around 200, and Linda decided in order to help me make the right food choices, the best thing was to not bring the food I shouldn't have into the house at all. I soon got used to my meals being high in low fat protein—chicken, fish, some beef or pork, and vegetables. Lots and lots of vegetables. Potatoes, rice, and pasta were totally off the table, literally. And she really went to the internet for her research on the best supplements to help with controlling blood sugar spikes.

This all happened in mid-summer, and I was still in the throes of dealing with the disease when Thanksgiving came around. Can you imagine NO dressing with your turkey at the family table? Topped off with green beans for desert. Yummy…..ok, not. But by this time I had seen how not staying on program and cheating on the diet made me feel sluggish, foggy, and have higher blood sugar readings. When I stayed on program, guess what—I felt better! It was amazing how smart I had become.

We had always believed in vitamins and aggressive supplementation but Linda's investigations found all kinds of new supplements to try out. And try them out we did. I took so many pills I think I rattled when I walked.

Well I had slowly gotten into a kind of rhythm in how I managed the treatment protocol—medications and diet—and was seeing my morning fasting readings slowly creep down. The joke was that if my Saturday morning reading was below 100 I could have my twice monthly pancake visit to IHOP (sugar-free syrup, please.) But it was working, slowly but surely.

And let me talk about what I see as a very, very important part of a three-pronged attack on diabetes and actually, pretty much any physical ailment. Modern medicine, when judiciously used, certainly plays a very important part, and a good healthy diet of proper foods and nutritional supplements only makes sense. But let's not forget about the spiritual side of what I call the Treatment Triangle. One's beliefs play a very significant part in healing our bodies, as well as the soul, spirit, etc. Prayer, meditation, Reiki, yoga, tai chi, whatever one finds good and healing to the soul I feel is good and healing to the body. I have no medical background to prove this. I just know that we increased the spiritual side of my treatment protocol and it worked for me. I think it amplified what my medications and diet had started, and that is when I really started seeing the tide turn in my favor.

Very soon my doctor's visit showed a good progress and he had me start cutting back on the insulin. From 30 units to 20 and my readings were still good, hovering around 100 or so for the morning fasting read. But I still needed the oral meds day and night to keep it on track. In other words it was better—good but not great, at least for us. My goal all along was to conquer this diabetes thing and get off medications entirely. I know not everyone shares this goal but it was my tape at the finish line and I set my mind on it. Day and night I wrote in my journal that I would cure the diabetes and not need medications.

Well I was feeling much better and seeing the readings stay constant or even lower, so I decreased the insulin on my own down to 10 units. With my readings still good, I told Linda, "It's time to see the doctor again and see what he says." When we told him I was down to 10 units a day he said the magic words we'd wanted to hear, "Ten units isn't much help so just quit the insulin and stay with your pills." Yippee! One less pinprick on my body, and part of the med-free goal was achieved.

I told the doctor about my med-free goal, and he said he keeps his patients on oral medications pretty much for life in order to manage their diabetes. For life I thought? Oh no, we are NOT having that. He said to keep on the meds and see him in a few months. So I continued my protocol—stricter diet, meditation, and journaling—but I wanted to see how not taking my oral medications for just a few weeks impacted the mix. When I went to see him he took the magic reading that diabetics go by, called AIC, and he said, "Wow, this is normal for a non-diabetic, much less someone with the disease." So he told me to stay off the oral meds and come back in a month. A month later and the AIC, plus my daily readings, were all in the normal ranges. He told me "It looks like your diabetes is in remission. You don't need to see me for now. Monitor your readings a few times a week, and come see me if it becomes a problem."

So while I cannot suggest everyone take this route to managing their diabetes, I can say this is what worked for me. I was very, very strict on my diet, especially at first, and faithfully augmented with supplements and followed my doctor's recommendations and medication protocol. I also added the spiritual side to my Treatment Triangle.

In closing, let me say this is never just one person's disease. I cannot say enough about the assistance, advice, and pushing (sometimes hard!) provided by my sweet wife, Linda. She made the journey much easier, and I would not have made it without her help. I hope this helps you as you read this, and I wish you peace and healing.

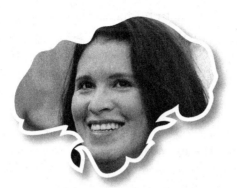

Gabi Pezo

Joy Designer, Art director and freelancer, Gabi Pezo is an Ecuadorian born laughter yoga and gibberish teacher, who loves to sing off key and is the mother of a 3 year-old soccer-obsessed toddler. Her first love for all things colorful and pretty started at age 4 when she opened her first Crayola crayon box. She went on to get her B.S in Mass Communications in Advertising and studied to become an Art Director.

As a multi-passionate being, her interest include spirituality, breath work and design. She discovered laughter yoga, the practice to laugh for no reason in 2007 and it was love at first laugh.

After a visit to an ashram in the Himalayas, her calling to be of service through Laughter Yoga became clear, and decided in 2012 to train with the creator of Laughter yoga, Dr. Madan Kataria and become a Laughter Teacher.

Gabi's commitment is to support people to take laughter and play seriously and teach them how to make it a useful and powerful tool to bring more joy and compassion into their lives, regardless of the circumstances they are facing.

She has also trained with humanitarian clowns in Ecuador and has participated in comedy and improv workshop in Dubai and USA, integrating all her experiences to develop unique and creative workshops for her students in corporations and healing centers in the Middle East.

Contact Gabi:

www.gabpezo.strikingly.com

✉ **gabpezo@gmail.com**

𝐟 **facebook.com/gabsterina.joy**

CHAPTER 10

MUNDAN (OR HOW MY PARADOXICAL DECISION LED ME TO WHOLENESS)

By Gabriela Pezo

The morning before I decided to shave my head, I wasn't able to stand up straight. I was dizzy, everything was spinning. And no, I was not drunk. Alcohol is not allowed in the ashram. There's also no internet, no real beds, and no privacy. This is my fourth morning waking up at the foothills of the Himalayas. And somehow I am starting to forget who I was before I arrived to this tiny ashram in Northern India.

The journey of how I found myself in this ashram in March of 2011 was unexpected. I had no conscious desire to go to an ashram or have a guru guide me through my spiritual path.

It all started in 2008 while living in Dubai. A gynecologist performed a pelvic ultrasound on my lower abdomen. "Well," she said, "you have PCOS, Polycystic Ovary Syndrome." PCOS is a health issue that affects a woman's hormones levels causing problems with periods and affecting ovulation. I knew this, so it was no news to me. I had been diagnosed with this in 2005 just after getting married but was told this was nothing to worry about and that it was quite common in women nowadays. "You do know what this means, right? You are not going to be able to have children."

She began interrogating me about my symptoms. I had none, except for the difficulty to lose weight. Still through all her questions, I was now clearly troubled at the thought of not been able to have children. All I could hear was: "You are not going to be able to have children."

Soon after the diagnosis my menstrual cycle became irregular and delayed. I was now experiencing one of the main symptoms of PCOS.

Apparently, the diagnosis was right. I was ill and had the symptoms to prove it.

In 2008, I confided in my best friend about this diagnosis and what the doctor had said. She was one of the only people that knew how scared and sad I was at this not-being-able-to-have-kids fiasco. "Don't tell anyone," she said. "No need to focus your energy to this or attract the pity of those who cannot help you." This is one of the wisest pieces of advice anyone has ever told me. She also suggested I look into the body-mind connection and find out what negative thought was creating this syndrome in my body. Her suggestion was: Breathwork-Rebirthing. Breathwork-Rebirthing is a powerful type of breathing where you lie down and start to breathe in a continuous and circular way. Since you are not moving, the energy accumulates in the body and the subconscious mind comes to the conscious mind, and you can deal with whatever you need to deal with: anger, sadness, guilt, etc.

I followed the advice and started to have regular breathwork sessions at least once a week. Every session was an hour long and each one of them was eye-opening and cathartic.

After a year of sessions, I was told that PCOS had disappeared from my body. (YAY!) I was really grateful about this and relieved that my body was back to normal. But there was still some issue in my subconscious mind that was standing in the way of me getting pregnant.

That year, I was invited to go to a workshop taught by Sondra Ray. I was in Miami, and my breathworker, who was extremely close to her, invited me and insisted that I must attend this workshop. Sondra is the mother of breathwork-rebirthing, a healer and spiritual teacher who has traveled the world over teaching people how to liberate themselves from the ego through the breath. I had read about her in a book and so I was excited to meet her.

As I entered the room where they held the workshop, I saw an altar all the way in the back. I walked towards it and saw a beautifully framed picture of a man with dark hair, with really strong and penetrating eyes. His hair all messy, and he was looking away from the camera. He looked like a handsome cavemen, so rustic, serious and his gaze like he was not just there but in another dimension. I later found out this was BABAJI, the mahavatar from the Himalayas. A mahavatar is a being that is not born of a woman. He materialized his body directly from God, the Source, the universe, or whatever you want to call the energy that started the world. Babaji left his body in 1984. Sondra told me she takes people to his ashram every spring for the divine mother festival. I knew I was meant to go to this place. I just couldn't stop thinking about this man in the picture. I was scared of him and at the same time attracted to his energy, the stories around him, his power.

By then, although my physical health was better, I felt like I wasn't good enough to be a mother, give birth to a child, or raise one. I didn't know why I had these thoughts. But the idea of being pregnant scared me. It was so scary that even though PCOS was long gone from my body, I still couldn't get pregnant.

In 2011, I started avoiding my reflection in the mirror. I just didn't like what I saw: a failed, insecure, ashamed, ugly woman. I avoided the mirror at all cost. I even brushed my teeth looking always down to the sink. And just as I started having these feelings about myself and my reflection, my periods were late AGAIN!

So the day before I had my head shaved in the ashram, I felt dizzy because of my fear of looking uglier, of feeling less feminine that what I already felt.

The thought of have my hair cut so short triggered a painful memory of my first haircut. I was five years old, and my dad took me to the salon to get my haircut. It was so short, and I hated it. I loved my long hair and my pigtails. I thought my hair made me beautiful and made me a girl. But because both my parents were busy working all the time, they decided to get me a low maintenance haircut. I am sure they meant no harm, but the action had a deep impact on me.

I had very short haircut until I was 11, so short people started confusing me for a boy when wearing pants or t-shirts. My mom wasn't very feminine herself, and as I said before, she was working ALL THE TIME. I knew I was a girl, but I was really angry when people thought I was a boy. And because of this, I thought of myself as an ugly duckling. I had equated long hair with beauty and being feminine.

So the idea of having my head shaved brought the thought that I will look so ugly and not feminine. And femininity was my struggle. That's why I had cysts and why these were in my ovaries, the vessels of feminine creative power.

Head shaving, or mundan, is a very powerful practice that signifies surrendering to the divine and letting go of all attachments. Our guru considered it a cleansing and healing practice that should be practiced by those who are serious about being liberated from their past.

The morning I shaved my head, the group I was with walked down to the river. I knelt down in front of the barber and placed the banana leaf on the ground to collect the falling hair. My husband held my hand throughout the ritual, and as the barber cut my hair from the root with the blade on my scalp, everyone at the ceremony started chanting, "Om namah shivaya," the maha mantra. Om namah shivaya means I honor the divinity within myself.

As I saw my hair dark, curly hair falling on the banana leaf, I felt warm tears rolling down my face. First, I felt deep sorrow and sadness that penetrated my heart and made me weep inconsolably. Memories from the day when they cut my hair as a child appeared in my mind, and I felt the emotions through my body. I felt as that part of me was leaving along with many other bits of garbage I had held on to. I was surrendering completely to God, to his will. I was placing my faith in him. Whatever was to happen, would happen. And as I let it all out, I felt an immense joy in my heart, indescribable joy. I started crying and laughing at the same time. But it didn't sound like my usual laugh, it was the laugh of a little girl, innocent and sweet.

It was done. I touched my bald head. I felt relieved. I picked up the banana leaf with all my long hair on top. I released it into the river nearby and waved good-bye.

I touched the back of my head and I felt as if I was a newborn: fragile, naked, and totally exposed.

I picked up the mirror. My reflection revealed a pale scalp; it needed some serious tanning. As I caught a glimpse of my face, I could see how big and bright my eyes were. I examined all of my face: my big strong cheekbones, my fat juicy lips, my strong chin. I was able to really see myself (maybe for the first time). It wasn't who I thought I was or who people thought I was but my true essence. The old feelings of rejection and disgust were simply gone.

The guru's advice is to keep the head shaven for nine months. I decided to do that. I was given a secret mantra to help me in the way I perceived myself as a woman, restore my creative feminine power, and eliminate the thought that I am not good enough to be a mother.

When I returned home, I dealt with what people said about me. Some thought I had cancer. My dad reacted as If I had joined a satanic cult. Children would point at me on the streets, horrified at the sight of me; men and women would stop me to tell me how beautiful I looked. All I knew was how comfortable I felt in my own skin.

After eight months, I decided I no longer needed to shave my head. I had no issues with seeing myself in the mirror. My periods went back to normal. Just before I decided to stop shaving I thought, "WHAT IF I DO GET PREGNANT? What if I do allow this to happen? Would it really be that bad? Would I really mess it up?" The questions didn't bring up fear, and I thought, "Maybe, I am good enough to be a mother. Maybe I will allow myself to be that." I had finally surrendered. This was just before Christmas 2011.

January came and I returned to India to train as a Laughter Yoga teacher. I also missed my period during my trip there. All I could think was, "Oh, God...NOT AGAIN! PCOS is back in my life." I also wasn't feeling all that well. I thought had caught a bug while in India. When I returned home from India, I was feeling worse and worse and decided to go see a doctor. I felt so ill that I thought it was serious. He ran many tests and discussed many possible scenarios.

When the results from all the test came in he said, "We can rule everything out. You are pregnant," but I thought I heard him say, "We can rule out that you are pregnant."

"I don't understand. Am I pregnant?"

He said again, "We can rule everything out. YOU ARE PREGNANT!"

We had this same conversation back and forth for at least 30 seconds until I realized what he was saying. I was going to be a mother. I was going to have a baby.

I was over the moon. My husband and I were both so happy; we cried that day when the doctor showed us our baby in an ultrasound. It was so crazy that I was nine weeks pregnant when we found out. All this time I had thought I was late because the PCOS had come back, and I thought that all of the digestive issues I had were because I had been in India. I went in the doctor's office that day expecting bad news and left feeling on cloud nine. Today we have a beautiful, active, and cheeky three year old running around our house, being our own little guru, helping us grow, much as we are doing for him.

I know my PCOS had to do with many issues surrounding my sacred femininity and holding that pain and sorrow from my first haircut. It was all intertwined in my mind somehow.

Through that part of my journey, I did breathwork regularly (I wish I did it more often nowadays). I also changed my diet (I was a vegan for a year), and became active (I ran a 10k and a half marathon). All of that supported me. But for me, my trip to the ashram in India completely transformed my life and who I thought I was. The spiritual practices really supported me: chanting, mediating, surrendering. But most importantly, shaving my head was the highlight of that part of my journey. Letting go of who I thought I was: someone who THOUGHT she wasn't good enough to be a mother, who didn't believe in her creative power to bring life or to deserve that, who didn't believe in her femininity. I became who I really am: me—a strong, powerful, and loving woman who knows I am more than just hair.

CHAPTER 11

EXUBERANT. EMPOWERED. ECZEMA-FREE

By Carina Lipold, MA

In my early teenage years, I used to walk down the street and look at the people passing me with wonder: how could they be so happy and vibrant? Sitting in my classroom looking around, I saw all those healthy girls and boys whose only worry seemed to be which shoes to buy next and which boy or girl to invite on a date. How come everyone was so normal except me? "That's not fair," I used to think and started to wonder why I got all the bad stuff while my friends got away with anything.

Why can't I wear short sleeves in the summer? Why does sweating hurt? Why can't I eat anything I wanted?

If you saw me today you would never guess where I started.

I was born with an auto immune disease, called atopic dermatitis. It is a form of eczema that is extremely itchy, can cover certain areas of your whole body, and comes in relapses. My parents tried to keep me from scratching my wounds and wrapped my little fists in cotton— but even with your fists wrapped in cotton you can scratch yourself with the wrapped knuckles till you are bleeding. My parents tried everything to make me feel better: I remember taking chamomile baths and baths with a lot of other substitutes that were supposed to help, putting me on special diets, taking Bach flowers, going to acupuncture, getting the typical cortisone and cortisone replacement ointments. To keep it short: they tried everything, but nothing really helped long term.

In my early teenage years—like probably many other girls the same age—I became interested in weight loss diets. I remember the first diet I tried was called "grazing," where you eat small portions every two hours during the day. I extensively studied this diet with my cousin. We would copy the book, collect articles, and make our own weight loss folder which served as the bible we lived by. Trying the new recipes and the first time closely paying attention how food felt in my body, I didn't lose weight but gained insights into how food would make me feel. It was the start of becoming more aware when it came to food. I noticed that white bread made me feel (and look) worse, as well as there being things I could not digest but that were apparently so healthy, like apples. Over the years, I stopped following other peoples diet plans and started to create my own, feel-good diet that was perfect for me.

During this process I became close friends with a school colleague that had type 1 diabetes. Seeing her measuring her blood sugar daily and injecting insulin or eating sugar naturally made me curious what my blood sugar level was. So I tested mine from time to time, whenever she had enough new needles with her. What I noticed was that my blood sugar level was very different during different times during the day and varied lot depending on what food I had during the day. After some observation, I realized which foods made my blood sugar level spike and which foods kept it down.

When I started the "grazing," it was all about calorie counting and achieving a certain number per day. In order to achieve this specific calorie count at the end of the day, exercise became an integral part of my daily life. Movement was always an integral part of my life—but with different focuses during my life. As a child, I had to move as I simply had too much energy and could not sit still (which drove my parents crazy at times). So they signed me up for Karate and other courses which I enjoyed (they also signed me up for flute, which I truly hated as I had to sit still for hours to practice... I would just sit beside the window, look outside to observe the other kids and play some melodies as they came to my mind in order to make a sound and pretend I was "practicing."

A few years after the "grazing" phase, the focus shifted to shaping up and having better results in track and field. In my later teenage years it shifted to more awareness when I realized how great exercise made me feel, how much I enjoyed being in nature and running, feeling my heart pumping… sitting on my bike and listening to the sound of the tires on the asphalt that became more intense the faster I went… and how happy, relaxed and aligned I felt.

Those experiences with diet and exercise all helped me to gain a new awareness about myself and feel better—but when it came to my eczema, I would still break out big time in stressful situations, like when I left my grandparents, when I broke up from my first boyfriend, or for my big a-level exams. So what was I missing?

As I am writing my story, I am sitting in a raw café in Bali looking into a river valley full of lush green. Just one week ago I had to leave my chosen home, Malaysia, unexpectedly due to bureaucratic challenges. This meant handing over my company, finding replacements for my clients, selling my car, getting rid of my apartment, packing everything, and saying good bye to my friends. Ten years ago, I would have had a major outbreak—but this time? Nothing. I am sitting here with clear skin, not a single spot to see. So what brought me to my current state? I want to share with you my seven biggest lessons learned:

1. **I am not alone**

   Many years ago, when I was walking down the street, it seemed that I was the only one that had issues. As time passed, I learned that's just the outside that we see. Many more people have health issues than we think—we just don't know about it. If you would see me on the street today, you would probably never think that I have health issues that I am dealing with. Realizing this, realizing that we are not alone… realizing that I was not alone, was a big step. You often can't see if someone has diabetes, an auto immune disease, or others. So don't assume.

2. **The Power of goal setting and visualization**

   In university, we had a great guest lecturer who was actually an alumnus of our university and a young and super successful entrepreneur. In his sessions he not only shared about the subject he was teaching, he also shared how he actually looks at life and how he became the person he is. Very powerful! One of the ideas he shared was to visualize where we see ourselves at 60 years old: what we see, hear, and feel. When we look back: what have we experienced? What kind of life do we want to look back at? It's a very powerful visualization that connects you to what really matters in your life. So I went back home and took this little booklet and started to write... and draw the picture that I had in mind, because I am a very visual person. Suddenly, all was what I wanted and my purpose in life was clear for me. From there, I set goals that are in line with my values and really inspired me and still do.

   A nice quote from Tony Robbins says: "People are not lazy. They simply have impotent goals—that is goals that do not inspire them." So when you pick your goals, make sure they are connected to your values, your deepest dream. Best test: if you feel so exciting writing them– then that's a great goal for you.

3. **The danger of energy vampires and the power of great friends**

   There are people that suck your energy and leave you feeling drained, and people that give you energy. I love to call the energy suckers energy vampires. We all have such people in our lives and they drain us by telling us that our plans are not going to work out or simply being negative. But how many people do you have that support your ideas—no matter how crazy they might seem at first? Surround yourself with people who believe in you and your ideas—they will bring you forward.

   Minimize contact with people who try to distract you—the energy vampires. Sadly, those people are often family and close friends. Of course you cannot remove them from your life, but you can limit the time you spend with them. It might be hard in the beginning, but once you see the success, it will bring you forward. At one point in my life I made a hard decision: I let go of some friends and limited the time spent with others and started to surround myself with people that give me energy. The effect was amazing!

4. **The circle of influence**

I love this one as it saves you so much energy that you can use for something else—something that makes you happy! And it's so simple! Only worry about what is in your circle of influence. Often I see people worrying about the bad behavior of other people, being angry about the traffic or politics, complaining about the horrible situation at their job. Well, we all have two options: Change something or accept and let go! Therefore ask yourself: Is the situation you feel bad about something you can change? If yes, how? If no—accept and let go. This is one of the reasons why I am not interested in politics.

5. **Move away from Black & White Thinking—find your own way**

We are in a very rule based culture. We judge everything as right or wrong. Everything is either black or white. I have always followed what I learned at university, the advice I received from experts... but my body started to really change and transform once I moved away from black and white thinking and found my own approach to nutrition, exercise, and other things. As I have a raw food business, people I meet are always shocked when they see me with cooked food or, even more, if they see me having a coffee. Often the perception is that if you do something, you have to do it perfect—but we are not looking for perfection... we are looking for what is good for us individually.

6. **Be mindful**

Our mind is often either in the past or in the future and being in the present moment can sometimes be hard to achieve—for me included. Meditation and mindfulness training helps us to generate more of those truly "present" moments and see life with all the bright colors it has.

During my first job, I heard about the 8 week mindfulness training and all the areas of life it would influence. So I went for it, and I am still very glad I did. Because our monkey mind doesn't get better as we grow older—it gets worse. Being able to control your mind and consciously turn all your thoughts on and off, or at least minimize them, is a great tool that will, first of all, make you more relaxed and happy and then everything in your life becomes easier: relationships, work, challenges. As you are not distracted, you can focus on what would be a real solution to a problem. Most ideas and solutions I have had were in such mindful moments. I am still far from perfect—but I'm getting better every day. Many people make meditation seem so easy... but you have to work for it, it's like training a muscle... only through repetition will it get stronger.

7. **Be grateful!**

Think at least once a day what you are grateful for in your life—it's a powerful habit. Personally, every night before I go to sleep, I reflect about the day. It started 10 years ago with 3 things I did well today—and that was really hard for me at this time because I didn't believe I did anything right. But I had committed to it, and eventually, I found more and more things I could write down. I then extended it and wrote down what external things I am grateful for—for example the nice sunshine, that my neighbor passed by out of the blue just to hand me a piece of cake, etc. Later, I also started to look at the things that I didn't do well, analyzed them, and mentally noted the lessons learned. One example would have been a negative reaction toward my friend: Why did I react this way? What triggered my bad behavior? How could I make it better next time? Some people also like to journal and write their experiences, observations, reflections, and lessons down. Choose whatever feels good for you.

These were my seven biggest lessons learned. In order to acquire the tools to help other people as well as continue the journey for myself, I did my Master's Degree in Health Management, got my Neuro-Linguistic Programming (NLP) Practitioner certification and various other certificates, such as Pilates Coach, and I worked on three continents in 4 different regions with beautiful people and organizations—all with the goal to inspire, empower, and transform.

Today, I see the eczema as an early warning system: when some spots appear, I know it is time to refocus on me again. I need to sleep more, decrease stress, be more mindful, and engage in activities that truly nurture me.

Through this journey and the lessons I learned, I could better deal with other health challenges that appeared later during my life. An example is the Hashimoto Thyroiditis I was diagnosed with—another auto immune disease. I do have to take my daily pills, but from reading other people's experiences, comparatively, I don't feel anything from it. Now I am embarking on my next journey: healing my thyroid gland and getting off my pills.

CHAPTER 12

HOW SELF-BELIEF, PERSISTENCE, AND SELF-LOVE CHANGED MY LIFE

By Dijana Green

When I was 34 years of age, I decided I needed to work on getting fitter and healthier before having children. I started a weight loss program and lost close to 40 kgs. I was going to the gym every day, six to seven times a week. I became a vegan vegetarian and life for me was wonderful. At 36 years of age, I gave birth to my first son, Aaron, followed by my daughter, Jessica Rose, and then my third child, Alexander. My three children were all born within a period of four years. During my pregnancies, I put on a lot of weight as I no longer exercised and ate far too much, however, I did lose most of my weight in between pregnancies without any problems.

As my eldest son turned four years of age, I left the corporate world and started my own international business. I started a technical services business implementing quality and food safety systems and offering training, process improvement, and nutritional services in the food industry. Being a qualified food scientist gave me the experience and knowledge to consult with food companies taking their quality and food safety to the next level.

I left the corporate world thinking I will have more time for my children but instead I embarked on a different adventure, an adventure that saw me reach peak success over night.

My international business was growing in double digits every year which created more travel and distance between my family and I. As a result, my marriage broke down and my health took a turn from operating at optimum health to becoming extremely stressed and unhappy.

My health problems were not so easy to diagnose. I went to see many doctors and had many tests, however, nothing was conclusive and nothing could explain what was happening to me.

I could no longer lose weight; my moods became inconsistent; I became unhappy, dissatisfied, always feeling cramps and pains in my stomach, bloating, constantly feeling tired, troubles digesting which all proved to be too difficult to diagnose and to pinpoint what was wrong with me.

I had no choice and from sheer desperation, I started listening to my body and started to do what felt right and self-healing. I started to analyze how I felt after eating certain food products and worked out very early in the process I could not digest starch, gluten, beans, pulses, and legumes.

Even though I knew eating these products made me feel unwell and uncomfortable, I did not know why. I never experienced this before so trying to work out what was wrong with me felt impossible.

I started to seek assistance from health practitioners such as naturopaths, iridologists, Bowen therapists, Ayurveda specialists, fasting and detox experts, and I even tried going raw. It all started to help, but I was still unsure of the root cause and what was making me feel so unwell after I would consume food products. It got to the point that whatever I would eat would made me feel unwell, uncomfortable, and bloated. Even exercising every day for an hour, working out at the gym, and working with a personal trainer would not shift any weight.

I started to grow tired of my illness and felt helpless on most occasions. A very good friend of mine was visiting a health clinic frequently in Thailand. He started to tell me all about his experience and how great it was. I wanted to go to the health clinic myself and determine if it would help me. My only problem was time and leaving the children and my business for twelve days.

Another twelve months passed and I continued to stress about my marriage breakdown and got busier with work before I decided enough was enough and if I don't place my health first I will not be alive long enough to support my children and see them grow up.

This gave me enough courage to book my first twelve days at the Spa Resort in Chang Mai Thailand. I was not sure if I could do the trip alone so a dear friend of mine Amanda Heather came along with me for support and encouragement.

I remember arriving on the first day crying and being afraid of how I would cope with no phone or computer and with being so far away from my children. The thought of relaxing and unwinding scared me. I did not know how to relax and unwind. I must say, after I got through my first day, I fell in love with the Spa Resort and then started to wonder what would I do when it was time to leave.

I woke up every morning and went to meditation classes, followed by yoga, then to start my morning colonics. I did two lots of colonic irrigations every day. Looking back now, I can say it was the best thing I ever did for my healing process. I fasted for seven days where I did not eat anything, and all of a sudden, I was feeling much better with no more sore stomach, bloating, or trouble digesting. Every day, I had a variety of spa treatments such as body wraps, facials, saunas, and massages. The massages were a treat. During my stay I read books, watched DVDs and started to learn the impact food has on my body and how each body is different. What worked for others may not have worked for me and vice versa. I met wonderful teachers like Nicole Van Hattem and Sunny Griffin. Both these ladies were very inspiring and taught me so much about eating raw. I also met a wonderful yoga instructor Frans Captijn; he too was most inspiring. The teachers and advisors at the Spa Resort helped transform my life. I even managed to attend raw food cooking classes held by the resident chef.

My health finally started to improve, and I started transforming my mind and mindset. When I returned home, I changed my diet and shifted to mainly a plant based diet, ate raw produce, and stopped eating sugar, gluten, dairy, and processed foods. This is when I started eating whole foods, organic products, and started to love myself more.

My transformation made such an impact on me that six months later I planned another trip to the Spa Resort. I did take another good friend Dianna Solek with me as I knew the impact it would also make on her life. Returning to the Spa Resort gave me strength and the ability to discover new beliefs. My mindset was shifting, and I loved it. I was feeling better than I had for the last five years and did not want it to stop. During my second trip, I started to learn to respect myself and my body more and started to understand what my body wanted and was calling out for. I still did not know what was wrong with me but I knew I was starting to feel much better and lighter.

When I returned from the Spa Resort in Chang Mai Thailand, my behaviour back home changed and my confidence with self-caring and self-healing was growing at rapid knots. I started to discover this was me; this is what I believe in and what makes me happy.

My children asked me if they too could eat what I was eating as they want to be healthy like mummy. I was absolutely delighted. I started with cleaning out our pantry and designing meal plans and lunch boxes that included mostly organic food, if not all organic, whole foods, grains, nuts, juices, and smoothies. I no longer purchased food in a box, and my children were eating homemade food only. An additive free lifestyle which also extended to what we put on our skin and in our hair, and we even threw out our microwave. We were no longer eating chicken nuggets, pizzas, McDonald's, chocolate, lollipops, muesli bars, and ice cream. My children do not feel like they are missing out as they get to eat it all, however, it is made fresh at home using organic ingredients and no gluten, sugar, or dairy.

The impact this lifestyle change has had on my family with schooling, education, and sports has been nothing short of amazing and has been the reason it has become our ritual to eat well and live a holistic life.

My family and I no longer visit doctors or consume medicine; we eat well, exercise, and drink lots of water. We spend a great deal of our time outdoors soaking up the sun and keeping active.

Continuing to work on achieving optimum health, I engaged services of a new naturopath who has been my life saver. Domenic Comminsio identified that the stress in my life had caused my digestion and gut to shut down. He pointed out to me that I needed to add protein with all my meals in order to prevent burning out and over using my adrenal glands. Domenic identified that I have chronic irritable bowel syndrome (IBS), and that I am allergic to lactose and intolerant to soy, almonds, eggs, and gluten. Following my new rotating eating plan, which Domenic created for me, stopped a lot of pain and unhappiness. A rotating food plan identifies what your body has difficulties breaking down or cannot digest too much of at any one time so you rotate what you eat every three days and limit how much of certain foods you eat. This way you can still eat what you enjoy without suffering stomach cramps and bloating.

My naturopath is teaching me the benefits of mindfulness, meditation, eating additive free foods, sleeping, and being grateful. All the tools and techniques I am learning, I can teach my children and others who want to know.

It has been my children who have been active in organizing for me to run health workshops in their school, teaching other children what I teach them about health and wellbeing. It is the big hearts of my children that encourage me to help others, to not give in and follow but to challenge and probe. To ask questions, challenge the norm and understand how your body works and how you can self-heal. How self-care leads to self-love, happiness, and paying it forward.

At the age of 43 now I have a better understanding of why my body needs to reduce stress from my life, what I need to do to reduce the stress, what to do to feel good, how to eat well, rest well, be more composed, temperate, and balanced, and how to live a holistic natural, healthy, and rich life.

CHAPTER 13

MY PURIFYING LYMPH PROTOCOL: FREEING MY VOICE!

By Sara Sophia Eisenman

It all began when I decided to get serious about writing my memoir: a deep and vulnerable telling of a life born into mental illness and abuse, and how I rose from that painful birthright into a higher version of myself, designed to serve as a map for the reader to utilize on her own journey. I was gung ho to write, but as soon as I sat down to my trusty computer and attempted to tell the deeper portions of my tale, it was as though my body started to fall apart. Although my mind felt "ready" to tell my story, my body had a much different opinion.

Coincidentally (although we all know there is no such thing), my family of four had been simultaneously exposed to a nasty stomach virus, and we all spent several days with fevers and vomiting. However, while my children bounced back within a matter of just a few days, I continued to run a high fever and soon contracted a painful case of laryngitis. It felt as though someone had shoved a large, highly obtrusive lockbox into/around my larynx, and my voice was literally taken from me. This poignant metaphor, which occurred right as I was attempting to tell my deepest truths, did not escape my attention.

I still expected to rebound quickly, as I always have, eating a healthy diet of whole, organic, nutrient-dense foods and being aware of self-care. However as time went on, rather than getting better I was taking turns for the worse—or at least the weirder—as my voice returned but in its place my entire lymphatic system began to swell. The lymph nodes in my throat, armpit, and groin became inflamed and enlarged, and I still had the feeling of a "lockbox" in around my vocal chords and throat that made me feel Iike I couldn't swallow. I had a strawberry-sized lump on the side of my throat and another in my neck underneath the opposite ear that caused a persistent earache. In addition, I would gag easily and was suffering from nausea as my lymphatic system continued to register pain and imbalance. All of this prohibited me from eating much, and I began losing weight rapidly, devoid of appetite.

I began to worry that something was seriously wrong with me, even that I might be dying. I decided to undertake a protocol of purification and very deep listening to my body and being, to allow my intuition to guide me. I had a strong sense that the abusive paradigm that I grew up in was still somehow "living" in me, encoded in my cells, and generating a "hold" on my vocal chords and being in a way that was preventing me from telling my story. I felt it was time to work very diligently on cleansing/releasing this old energy that was no longer serving me, in order to clear the path for a new version of myself to be born.

In fact, I had been through this sort of energetic "death" process before, and I truly believe that many, if not all, of us are asked to "die" multiple times while still alive—shedding outdated versions of ourselves—in order to rise more deeply into our full truth and being. The very recognition that this happens was a comfort to me and allowed me to reduce any fear/attachment to outcome which I believe enabled and empowered me to heal.

Throughout this process, I was committed to allowing the highest good to be enacted. This "illness" was here to be my teacher, and it was my decision not to visit a medical doctor where it would likely be diagnosed and pathologized, but rather to view my symptoms as a roadmap to a higher version of myself, while being very open to receiving assistance and support from the many talented healers, if and when it organically presented. Thus, while I didn't "believe in" my symptoms, in the sense of wanting to name and categorize them as an "illness" (which would have perhaps crystalized and "locked" them into reality in a counterproductive way), I chose to honor them and listen to my body very deeply.

To undertake this process, I began taking very intense detoxification baths in which I would purposefully sweat. I turned off all artificial lighting, using only dim natural light or candlelight. I started by body brushing with a dry brush to stimulate my lymphatic system and promote healing. To facilitate a state of deep relaxation that allowed for physical catharsis and the chance to "tune in" to my body as well as nourish my body, I alternated between epsom salt, "real" salt, aluminum-free baking soda, and once a week would use an extremely potent ayurvedic "mustard bath" formula. I would allow beads of sweat and often tears to emerge on my face and roll down my cheeks and off my chin—that was my measure that deep release was taking place.

Each time I engaged in this process, I closed my eyes and asked to receive/witness whatever revelations my body wished to share with my conscious mind, intentionally creating a "bridge" between the two. At times, I received very detailed and precise information about which forms of nutrition to use in my healing process, while other times the information I received was much more energetic/spiritual in nature. Many times, the unfinished "stories" still housed in my body would present themselves for healing. I would find myself suddenly having an internal "argument" with a family member regarding a situation of years past that had not yet found resolution or feeling guilt/shame regarding a wrongdoing I perceived myself to have done long ago. Many times, these "stories" felt like they were associated with specific energy meridians of my body, which were blocked by uncleared energy. For example, one such "story" was associated with a blockage in the energy line from my heart space to my left hand.

I committed to taking full responsibility for whatever arose, and asked my body what I needed to do to process the energy fully and release/heal the "story," which often involved writing letters with words that needed to be spoken, clearing and reconnecting ancestral lines, and much more. I was very open to receiving support and had several highly talented, trusted energy workers spontaneously offer to clear my throat chakra and support my healing. Shamanic journeywork, facilitated by my husband and myself, was also key to my healing. It turns out that there was a soul part in my energy system who was still not "free" from the trauma that had taken place in my childhood. She believed that she would die if she told her story and needed love and healing. There was also a dramatic journey in which my lymphatic system, which had been basically energetically "blown out," was upgraded with liquid light and mapped onto the universal tree of life. There was also a point at which I was called, very fiercely, to stake a claim for my own healing and *command* (not ask) that it be so, to prevent me from simply fading into the night of this "death" process. (These profound healings are recounted in much greater detail in my forthcoming memoir.)

I was also guided to a very specific nutritional protocol, as follows: In the morning, I drank water with a tablespoon of apple cider vinegar and ingested several chunks of fresh raw ginger before eating a single thing. Some days, I similarly ingested chunks of raw garlic as well. Most mornings, I ate a whole, fresh, organic pineapple for breakfast, accompanied by a cup of organic chicken bone broth. For lunch, it was bone broth again with some very soft, well-cooked rice mixed with ghee, and dinner consisted of lean protein (chicken or fish) with greens and soft, starchy food such as boiled potatoes with butter. I supplemented with fresh pressed fruit juices and smoothies. All of my food had to be extremely well cooked and soft for me to tolerate it. I avoided coffee, almost all dairy, alcohol, red meat, and anything fried or acidic. I also used copious amounts of hot sauce in my food, ranging from the milder jalapeno peppers all the way up to the spiciest habanero sauce I could find. Thanks to a local Peruvian restaurant and its authentic cuisine, I was even introduced to a special pepper native to Peru that was the spiciest and most detoxifying yet. During the deepest portion of my detox, I consumed up to a whole bottle of habanero hot sauce per day, which both stimulated my digestive capacity and facilitated deep release.

As important as what I put in my body was what I put *on* it. I used copious amounts of castor oil on my throat, inside the affected ear (using a dropper and/or a cotton ball), and on the affected lymph nodes under my arms, applying several times per day and massaging the oil into the area. Once a week, I prepared an abdominal castor oil pack for my abdomen, and left it on overnight to support lymphatic healing. I also found an organic ginger and cayenne massage oil at my local health store and diligently massaged the affected areas with this as well. Lastly, I was guided by a friend to apply one drop of Young Living Frankencense oil, blended with a teaspoon of castor or other oil, to the throat area—and once I did that the lumps in my throat begin to noticeably shrink and normalize.

My appetite slowly returned, and the lumps in my neck and pain in my ear all but vanished. However, I then began having other troubling symptoms: dizziness, feeling faint, migraines, tingling in my extremities, and debilitating fatigue. My spiritual guides revealed that I had become anemic due to nutrient loss from the very intense purification/detoxification process and needed large amounts of a wide range of nutrients to recoup. It was very interesting to observe the tipping point of the pendulum swing between purification ("death") and the need for nourishment ("rebirth"), as I began to understand ever more deeply the complementarity of these twin processes. I began drinking large amounts of nutrient-dense organic smoothies containing beets, a wide variety of dark greens, and nourishing fruits, such as mango and banana. I focused on iron-rich seafoods such as oysters and salmon and iodine-rich seaweed, as well as whole cooked beets with plenty of butter. I also supplemented with Floradix, an all-natural iron supplement. Equally important, I committed to resting whenever I needed, even if it meant sleeping right in the middle of the day sometimes (it did!).

As of this writing, I am still doing all of the above and feeling so much better! I have had the strength and stamina to write over half of my book without return of the aforementioned symptoms, save the occasional "echo." I feel lighter and better in my body than I ever have, and my voice is now free to express itself in full—and I know it is because I truly listened and agreed to engage fully in my healing process from a standpoint of love and willingness rather than fear. Another key was being open to receive all forms of aligned "external" support, recognizing that this gift, too, begins in the universe within. I have the deepest gratitude for this miraculous universe that continues to amaze me every single day!

If the reader is so inclined to connect more deeply, this is the type of healing work in which my husband and I are thrilled and honored to support others.

With infinite love and gratitude,
Sara Sophia Eisenman

CHAPTER 14

THANKS MULTIPLE SCLEROSIS FOR ALLOWING ME TO HIT ROCK BOTTOM

By Rev. Sam Shelley

I was lying in the hospital bed unable to walk due to the numbness on the left side of my body. I was unable to use the bathroom and one eye was moving around uncontrollable and the other eye was blurry. I was lying there wondering what I did to deserve my latest health challenge. This was in the spring of 2004, after the worst migraine of my life had landed me in the hospital for several weeks.

During my time at the University of Pennsylvania Hospital, I had many medical tests. All my tests were coming back negative, yet a few tests suggested that I had multiple sclerosis (M.S.). When I viewed my brain MRI, I saw bright spots (M.S. lesions) along with the normal dark color of the brain, which created a whimsical Swiss cheese image. These "holes" in the brain are a sign of demyelination of the white matter of the brain, meaning protective sheaths around the nerves in my brain were damaged.

When I arrived at the rehab center, the social worker asked what I knew about M.S., and I told her not much. She came back with literature on the disease. This pamphlet made me feel even worse. It talked about how 80% of people diagnosed with M.S. end up in a wheelchair after ten years. I also read about how M.S. is the number one cause of disability among young adults—I was 37 years old when diagnosed. The neurologist at the rehab evaluated my mental state and ordered a psychiatric consultation. This psychiatrist adjusted my medication to help stop my crying spells.

After a few weeks, I was recovering and could walk 50 feet using a walker. When I could take care of all my basic needs, including feeding myself, going to the bathroom, etc., I was able to return home. When I arrived home another shock wave hit me. My home was not handicap accessible. Everything that I took for granted became an obstacle. The sidewalk leading to the front door had a slight uphill incline. The stairs, the coffee table, and the throw rugs throughout the house were impossible. I took my ability to walk for granted.

Every morning at home after rehab, I woke up in a mental state of dread. I was always wondering what else was going to go wrong (Before this hospital stay and rehab, I was diagnosed with bipolar, psoriasis, psoriatic arthritis, and migraines) or how I was going to function for the day. Will I be able to walk, swallow, go to the bathroom, or will I end up in a wheelchair?

After the M.S. diagnosis, I finally reached a point of being sick and tired of being sick and tired. I hit rock bottom with no way out, and I had no idea where to turn besides my team of doctors. The doctors' ideas to help heal me were by taking medicines to the point that I was up to 13 medications a day.

In 2010, I was a couch potato and I watched a lot of television. I would watch anything, and I found myself fascinated by ghost hunting shows. Although I had no idea if ghosts were real or fake, it was TV, and TV is scripted. One day I was on Twitter and saw a tweet from a ghost hunter from one of the TV shows. They tweeted about an upcoming event they were doing at Fort Mifflin in Philadelphia. I signed up for the event and when the day arrived, I put on my M.S. cooling vest. Because of M.S., I was very sensitive to heat and my body would shut down if I became overheated. I was able to explore the fort for about 90 minutes before the ice packs melted.

I saw events on the ghost hunt that I could not explain. I saw flashlights were going on and off by command. I sensed someone sitting next to me that I couldn't see. I became overwhelmed with a strong sense of dread.

I started to read a few books trying to understand my experiences on that summer evening. After several months, I read a book that discussed meditation. A benefit that immediately caught my attention was "inner peace." When I read those words, I immediately knew what I needed.

That night, I began a simple meditation practice. I didn't have a mediation teacher, and the book I was reading provided little advice on the subject. My easy practice had me sitting there for five minutes and not reacting or responding to my thoughts. Initially, this was hard, and my mind was telling me that I was wasting my time. My mind told me there were better things for me to do. I just had a feeling that a daily meditation would help me gain inner peace.

After a few weeks, sitting still during meditation became easier. After a month or two, my mind was growing quiet. I was seeing that inner peace could be my reality. By the third month of meditation, I was sitting for ten minutes in the morning and ten minutes in the evening. After one evening meditation, I heard a voice say "perfect spirit." I knew that was my answer and that my spirit was perfect. It was my damaged body and mind that was unwell. Then I had a deep knowing that "all is well," and all sense of fear about my health melted away.

I now see my M.S. diagnosis as a blessing. My inability to function forced me to watch a lot of television. Through a TV show, I went on a ghost hunting adventure. This ghost hunt led me to have paranormal experiences. These paranormal experiences led me to read a book about meditation. Through meditation I learned about my true self. When I finally realized that I was more than my thoughts is when I made a miraculous recovery. Today, I have no signs of the disease, need no medication, and no longer need a cane or walker.

It was unknown to me at the time, but I was taking a series of small steps to recover my health. If I had the mindset that meditation would reverse all my diseases, I would have failed—that is too big of a leap. Yet I took a small step with a simple meditation practice as a way to gain inner peace. As the Chinese philosopher Lao Tzu said, "The journey of a thousand miles begins with one step."

When I look back today on the past when I was lying in bed asking, "Why me?" and "What did I do to deserve these diseases? " Today, I say "Why not me? I'm a human just like everyone else, no one is exempt from their human experiences. "

I can see now that nothing was happening to me and everything was happening for my benefit. In addition to M.S., life gave me four other incurable diseases, and I had reached a point of "ENOUGH!" I was at rock bottom, and I had to be open to explore new ideas and venture away from the traditional medical system. A medical system that was maintaining the status quo -- with no cures.

The prominent Greek physician Galen of the Roman Empire once said, "The best doctor is not outside of you, for you are your best doctor. For this is your body, and you know it the best. "

Before my meditation practice, I didn't know my body too well. I had constant noise in my mind guessing how my body and my mind should behave. Through mediation I learned to quiet my mind, and when my mind became quieter, my intuitive voice became louder. This intuitive voice told me how to improve my health from all my conditions.

Everyone has this quiet intuitive voice but our loud noisy minds overshadow our intuition. We are not taught how to quiet the mind to increase the volume of natural intuition. I recommend that everyone has a simple daily meditation practice.

Here is my meditation practice:

1. Find a comfortable place with no interruptions to sit.
2. Dress comfortably.
3. Do not concern yourself with hand positions or breathing in a specific way.
4. Set a timer for two to five minutes to begin a meditation practice.
5. Close your eyes.
6. Relax!

When thoughts arise, do not react or respond to them. If you notice thoughts are grabbing your attention ask yourself: "What am I touching?" "What am I smelling?" "What am I hearing?" You want to engage the senses, for your senses are always in this moment, your thoughts are not in this moment. Your thoughts are reliving yesterday or guessing tomorrow. The more you are in this moment, the more inner peace you will discover.

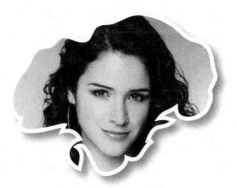

Paola Albo

Hi! My name is Paola and I'm proudly Mexican.

I've always knew that there was something else than the physical experience. Since I was a little girl, the interest and the abilities over the supernatural have been present in my life.

At 6 I had my first regression to my past lives, at 14 I started doing yoga and meditation. When I felt the calling to start my spiritual journey, the doors were magically opened for me to enter.

From that moment on, I've been preparing myself non-stop in different holistic therapies and energy healing, taking whatever information I could get, courses, workshops, certifications, all of them focused towards conscious development and inner work.

My life mission was revealed when I discovered that I could make people feel better with my words. So I started studying a degree in psychology with the purpose of complementing my holistic practice healing the symptoms from their roots.

At the moment I'm doing my certification as a Health Coach, a course in Family Constellations and giving therapies to people seeking a new path to health. My therapies are the result of integration of theta healing, reconnective healing, plus my degree in psychology and health coach, making and integrative approach to the wellbeing of the person. I've come to realize that the true master is inside ourselves, and everybody needs a different path and a personalized guidance.

I'm here to help you make this world a healthiest, happier and full of love.

Contact Paola

- 📞 **+55 2919 9222**
- Ⓢ **paoalbos**
- ✉️ **reprogramate.7@gmail.com**
- f **ReprogrAmate con Paola Albo – facebook.com/salud2015.P**
- 📷 **@Soy_Paoalbo**
- 🐦 **@Paoalbo**
- 📍 **@Paoalbo**

CHAPTER 15

HUNGRY FOR LOVE

By Paola Albo

Today I begin a new era, finally being able to feel the beats of a heart willing to live.

This is my story.

Since the day I was born until I was 5, I experienced the feeling of living in a bubble, where everything was beautiful and pink. Inside that bubble I felt completely safe, nothing bad ever happened. There was no conflict, no confrontations, no sadness, no tears, and everything was perfect in appearance. I never learned to ask for help. Why would I? My family was perfect, and I wanted to belong.

At the age of 6, even though to me my parents appeared to be happy, they were getting a divorce. It must have been so painful that my little-self buried the memory and the experience somewhere deep down in my subconscious. I didn't know it would take 16 years until it all came back for me to process it. At the time, a special journey started, a journey within, to save that little girl inside of my head who desperately fantasized about keeping her parents together. The relationship with my dad grew distant while the codependency with my mother grew stronger.

When I turned 15, my sister told us she wanted to be an artist. Her talent as a singer evolved, and she started getting recognition and opportunities. Family and friends started talking about her amazing voice and charisma. Everybody loved her and so did I. From singing at family reunions to big theaters and plays, I went from being her sister to being her shadow. I felt so tiny in comparison. No matter what I did, I realized that my efforts were in vain. Nobody had eyes for me. It was all about her.

"I must be doing something wrong," I thought, "I'm not good enough".

The idea of not being good enough became an obsession until resentment and anger towards my family became a daily emotional leitmotif. However, I never said anything and managed to keep all my pain and the guilt growing inside my head.

In high school, my grades were excellent from the get go. I finally found a spot in which I could excel and be visible, and I could feel the sweetness of perfection that I needed. I finally got my father's attention, but I was still invisible to the rest of the world.

"Here I am!" but no one else noticed me.

Getting perfect grades was an easy task for me, so there was no room for errors. My obsession with perfection led me to loneliness and humiliation. The better the grades, the worst the bullying and rejection. Due to the fact that I was feeling so depressed, I barely managed to finish high school.

Every night I lit incense, put on soothing music, and sat down to meditate in my room, knowing that I would find the peace and joy that I couldn't find on the outside. Meditation was a healing energy that made me remember, in little glimpses, my true essence... that being of light that gave me the energy I needed to hold on one more day.

I started practicing yoga and meditation at 14. I've always been sensitive to extra sensory phenomenon, and a year later, I felt the inner calling to keep going on that deep spiritual path. Courses, workshops, books, and people started crossing my way and I understood: the universe was showing me the way, and I followed it.

As this spirituality became a very important part of my lifestyle, my body started rejecting meat, so I became a vegetarian.

Only one month after finishing high school, the bill from all the feelings that I tried so hard to hide arrived. My mother's second divorce fired the beginning of my disease. We were looking for a new home, and at the same time, I got casted to host a TV show that was going to be filmed on a beach. I wanted to look good in a bikini, so I started working out seven days a week and made little adjustments to my diet.

I only lost five pounds, but it made people turn around. I started receiving the attention I'd been looking for and getting the motivation to look and feel better. I started classifying food by "good" and "bad" according to the amount of calories it had, and the obsession grew. It didn't matter how healthy or little I ate, they were too many calories in it. I was getting through the day with one apple and lots of water.

The change was unnoticeable to me. Suddenly, I was the puppet of a voice inside my head. Every time I fantasized about stopping that "little" obsession, it mocked me and blew me away. My light went off, I was in the darkness, paralyzed, scared, and barely breathing.

I understood hate. I wanted to kill myself for being fat. Every night the voice started yelling at me and I begged God to take me away, and every morning I was exhausted, but looking at myself in the mirror and seeing my bones made me think it was all worth it, so I kept going.

One day, after over purging myself for a whole weekend because I dared to eat an extra apple, I caused a deep dehydration that guaranteed me entrance to a special clinic for eating disorders. I was terrified, but there was no other way out.

After a week in the clinic without any contact from the outside world and under vigilant 24/7 observation, I understood that the problem was not the food, it was everything deep down, (as is with a lot of other diseases). I was inside four walls with a lot of time to think, so I didn't have another choice but to start truly looking at myself and my wounds.

I took the responsibility of my own recovery without giving power to anything outside myself. For the first time in 18 months, I heard my soul talking again.

"You are in your hands" — my soul whispered. And I held that.

This affirmation was the key to my recovery because every time I relapsed and lost weight, I remembered that there wasn't a safer place to be than my own hands.

It was really tough to be in the clinic, so I got out feeling like if I stayed I was going to lose my mind. As soon as I left, I bought myself an engagement ring and promised to myself never to go back there. I also made a promise that once I got strong enough, I would help lots of people to heal and teach them how to nourish their body and soul and not to wait until their body starts to scream for help.

I continued my recovery outside the clinic supported by a group of doctors. Even though I relapsed, the fear of going back to the clinic was so strong that I actually used it in my favor and the fear kept me moving forward.

Saying that the journey was easy would be a lie. It was hard and painful but worth every step. I could've waited to be rescued for 20 years, but that wasn't going to happen. I took a deep breath and took the first step. I realize now that the hardest thing is to start.

I accepted that I needed help to change my mindset. I took my therapy seriously and gave myself to the process as if my life depended on the capacity to ask for and accept help. I finally let all of the feelings out that I'd been keeping and opened my heart. Having professional help guide me through a fascinating journey to the depths of my being helped me understand a lot.

As soon as I could return to exercise, I did it, not as a means to lose weight, but as a way to channel stress and unwanted feelings in a healthy way. I was fascinated with myself for becoming the person I always wanted to be, so I became very selective with everything that affected my life: food, hobbies, people, thoughts, feelings, etc. This way I started nourishing not only my body but my soul. I regained contact with nature, meditation, and alternative therapies which made me remember what happiness is.

Motivated by the promise I had made of helping others, I started studying psychology and began my certification as a health coach. With new information and knowledge, plus my own experience, I am keeping good on my promise.

That being said, I know there is a reason why you are reading this. Because you know what? Divine timing does exist. Maybe this is the signal you were waiting for to start moving. No matter how hard it might seem DON'T give up. You will find a way because you are worthy. You are already stronger than you think. You just have to remember who you really are. These are the steps that helped me:

Start. That is the secret. Take the first step and give yourself to it. As long as you give yourself to the process of healing, the doors of your inner world will open showing you the road to follow so you can reach the second step.

Follow the road. You'll find days when the sun won't come up, but there will be lots of days also when you'll find that the light will come to you in all directions easing the anguish and awakening your being. Use those days to fill yourself up with hope.

Be patient. The only way to make it is by trial and error. So keep trying, over and over again, because you don't know at what point you will finally get to knock on the door that will lead you to a better place. Each day you don't reach the door, breathe and start again while always remembering God is holding your hand for every step.

Take a deep breath and feel. The only thing stronger than your mind is the power inside your heart—that voice that barely whispers and encourages you to try one more time, because every day is a new beginning.

It is time.

Unlock and open the doors. Give up being a victim and turn into a conqueror by asking yourself the "what for," not just remaining angry about the "why." Don't wait any longer. There is no day like today.

Ask for help, take action, and break the silence.

YOU ARE IN YOUR HANDS.

Light, peace, and love.

By the way, I am grateful for the anorexia, because in a deep act of love, it brought me back to life.

CHAPTER 16

10 MATCHES
By Agnieszka Zwierzynksa

I'm not writing this story to look for sympathy. I am writing this story to show every woman and girl that every struggle in life can be won, that everything depends on your mindset and how strong you are inside. It's about motivation. I call it fighting.

I grew up in a wealthy family in a large city in the northern part of Poland. I have one younger sister. My first memory is of my mum bringing my sister home from the hospital after she was born. The second was when she was learning to walk. And the third, when my grandmum threw away the leather belts my dad used to hit us with when we weren't listening. My later memories are of blood everywhere and running away from home.

My mum was 16 years old when she had me. She was very young. My dad was 22. My mum came from a family where her dad left her, her four siblings, and her mum and ran off with another woman. She didn't have any support, so she got married to my dad when she was 16.

My dad was a smart man. My granddad on my father's side was very wealthy; he owned a lot of land and property within our city and he helped my dad build a house in 1993. In that same year, my parent's opened a large pub with a small restaurant. It was a "gold" business with incredible income.

As far back as I can remember, my dad was always threatening my mum. She always had marks on her body and face, and it always seemed there was dried blood somewhere. Up until I was 14 years old, she tried to divorce him probably 20 times. Even though her family supported her in this, she always came back to him. Always. She would say that she couldn't give us anything on her own.

Finally, she couldn't handle it anymore. She started drinking so she wouldn't feel what he was doing to her. At 14, I became the managing director for two thriving businesses, because my dad also became a full-time alcoholic. I can't remember much of what was happening with my sister at this time. She was mostly in the care of my auntie. I didn't know anything about running a business. The only people around me were trying to use me to get more for themselves. Nobody cared about us—just about how much money they could get with my parents not available. It was hell. My childhood was one of domestic violence. I don't know what a childhood is at all.

"10 Matches" was how my father taught my sister and me to clean the pub (which was almost always open, only closing to be cleaned). After we'd work, he'd say, "I hid 10 matches in places that should have been cleaned. If I walk around and don't find any matches remaining, it means you did a good job. If I find matches, it means you are going to do it again." I am now thankful to my dad for this lesson.

At 18, I got pregnant by a boy from my neighborhood, one I knew well from playing together as children at the playground. I thought we would always be in love. However, it very quickly became a nightmare. He started hitting me in my fourth month of pregnancy. My parents didn't like him, and they weren't happy about my pregnancy. They wanted me to get an education and, one day, take over the family business. My father kicked me out of the house, so I was mostly on my own since the father of my child didn't care about me. I lived with my grandmum who, along with my mum, helped me. I began working in a tax-council office on a school project. I don't remember much from that time.

In my ninth month, I still looked like I was in the beginning stages of pregnancy with a very small bump. Finally, on May 19, my son, Wiktor, was born. My father came to the hospital and begged me to come back home, but I said no. After two months, my mum asked me the same question, explaining that they wanted me to finish high school and continue my studies.

So I moved back home. My father promised to stop drinking. He stopped for a year before starting again, and we were back to our "normal"—an alcoholic father and me going to school, running a business, and raising a one year old. I did have support from my auntie who took care of my son for me. I also had about ten men interested in me at this time, but they were all interested in just the money that our business made. It became year after year of the same thing.

Between my two alcoholic parents, we had an ambulance at our house five times, along with private nurses to care for my ailing father. Again, it was hell. And the worst part was that my son was witnessing it all. It's very hard to write about, even now. My mum spent time at private rehab facilities and everything fell on my shoulders because my sister was too young.

Somehow, I finished high school and went on to university where I studied management and marketing, even though that wasn't my interest; it was easy to continue on with it after high school. I was always interested in architecture or photography. My passion was dancing, and I danced for a couple of years, but my father said I needed to learn skills. No time for passions.

At 27, I moved to Northern Ireland. I didn't see a future for my son living like we were with my father using us all the time. We worked so that he could drink and have fun; he didn't care about us at all. It was a big shock, but I went from business owner to a general operator in a window fabric factory. It was refreshing to wake up and realize no one was shouting or drinking, yet there was a roof over mine and my son's heads. That was what kept me going.

After working for four months, I lost my job due to layoffs. I was the first to be laid off since I had to come in late in order to drop my son off at school in the morning. I went four weeks without work, waking up every day and searching, while also supporting my brother-in-law who was searching for work as well. I finally found work as a cleaner during the day and as a dishwasher in a restaurant at night. I had a friend that cared for my son at night while I worked.

Years later, I was still working all the time. I was about to turn 30 and felt like the last whistle was about to blow on my chance for another child, so I got pregnant. My then-partner turned out to be the same as my father, but he concentrated on my son and was very bad to him. After a year, I left him. Again, I was doing all the hard work to maintain my family, but this time with two children.

Soon after, I was involved in a car accident. I was driving down a very steep hill in the middle of the night when my car started sliding and nearly hit a tree. My life was saved by a road sign and a fence. (Then about a year later, I had another small crash.) I was not lucky with cars at this stage of my life. I was in such a state of shock when I went to work the next day. I went to the hospital with neck and sciatica pain two days later, but they treated me like I was nuts for coming in two days after the accident. They didn't do any x-rays or MRIs to check on me.

My worst pain began a week after the accident. I had to stay in bed; if it wasn't for my mother, the kids wouldn't have even made it to school. I would crawl out of bed, crying in pain, every morning just to get to the bathroom. This went on for two weeks. I finally started on painkillers and, later, on physical therapy.

At my own expense, I had x-rays and an MRI done and found out that two of my disks had shifted and were touching nerves. Whenever the disks came in contact with the nerves I would feel a painful current go from my head to my big toe. My physiotherapist did what he could, but twice there were times when I couldn't do a single thing he asked of me. I tried group therapy but was excluded after five minutes when he told everyone to lie on their backs, which created the worst pain for me. My doctor then directed me to do individual therapy.

I also had to return to work. My disability benefits ended, but my kids still needed to eat. I needed a huge amount of medication to even function on a daily basis: codeine, tramal, acetaminophen, and anything else that was on hand. I was taking so much medication, if I went out for a drink with friends (at least people who I thought were friends at the time), I couldn't feel my legs. That amount of pain meds and one or two drinks were nearly killing me. Even still, I spent almost every weekend with a glass of whiskey in my hand; destroying my body even more week after week. My health was starting to completely fail, and I was also struggling with anxiety and depression. One day, I had to decide whether to give up or keep going. My heart made the decision, and day-by-day, I gave up cigarettes, alcohol, drugs, and my weekend lifestyle. I was glad that I had my mum and my kids with me while I went through those times. My mum, trying to prove how I strong I was, told me, "When you came into this world, the first injection the doctor gave you, you broke the needle because you were so tough."

After all I went though, I think my back pain was nothing compared to the pain I was dealing with internally. I have been learning how to deal with my past, but from time to time the memories still come back. I still have signs from the domestic abuse—one eye is permanently destroyed and my nose has been broken a couple of times. I plan to have surgery to correct this one day.

Last year was one of the worst of my life, because I was dealing with anxiety and depression due to a loss of money. Since then, I have met a wonderful woman who became my business mentor. She did an exercise with me where she showed me a list, which included: family, money, health, beauty, etc. She asked me what was most important and what had I lost. She also gave me examples of people who had lost millions, but yet still survived. We tend to think that our current situation is the worst it can be, but it is not truly like that. She showed me how many struggles people all over the world are facing.

At 34 years old, I now know that the worst part of my life was the violence I faced. I still have a lot to overcome, and I still have a lot of insecurities in regards to my relations with men. But I don't want to be on my own forever. I like to be in love; I'd like to share my life with another person.

I have met some amazing people who motivate me, even if they don't know it. After I started my business, I met a man who would always help me out. He taught me a lot, and I appreciate it. I also met two wonderful women who helped me understand things I previously couldn't understand. And I finally met the man of my dreams—but that is a long story, maybe one for another book. I am still not sure if he feels the same about me, but there is hope.

The main message I want to share with all women is that you should never give up. Good things come from hard word and faith. Faith will keep you alive. My kids were my motivation.

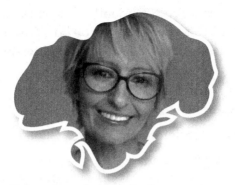

Christine Marmoy

Mom of 4, 46 years old.......and Christine Marmoy still wears a size 0!

After being a vegetarian all her life, and raw and vegan for the past 3 years, she became very sick. Until she discovered the reason: Food Allergies: Cross Reactivity with Pollen!

Allergies can cause many symptoms, 2 of the main ones being a bloated feeling or being overweight. While learning to work around her allergies, Christine came to understand the reason for her constantly bloated stomach, the very problem she couldn't seem to get rid of.

If you have food sensitivity, you have an inflammation and if you do, then your belly won't go away through diet and exercise alone. You need a full reset and that's just what Christine does.

In order to help other women regain control over their own body and feel healthy and sexy inside and out, she created a magazine called Raw & More which is available on all phones and computers along with having a huge community of followers on Facebook. She has developed specific programs to help anybody to slim down their waist using sound nutrition and supplements and adequate exercise techniques which everybody can easily perform.

Christine is a Certified Ashtanga Yoga instructor, a licensed Personal Trainer (NASM) as well as holding an MBA. She is currently studying Nutritional Endocrinology.

Get started with her FREE "Smoothies for a Beautiful YOU" where you'll find succulent recipes and tips on how to sculpt your new body today—**www.rawandmoremag.com/smoothies-beautiful-you**.

Contact Christine:

www.rawandmoremag.com

✉ **christine@rawandmoremag.com**

f **facebook.com/rawmom**

CHAPTER 17

NO THANKS! I DON'T WANT A WHEELCHAIR

by Christine Marmoy

It was another beautiful day in Barcelona, the little region of Spain which is well-known for its microclimate; just 65 days of rain and 300 days of full sunshine from morning to evening. With a sea view from my apartment and the cliffs to hike, what more could I have asked for?

One night, I began to experience a pinching pain in my right leg, although I didn't really pay much attention to it at that time; we were walking a lot so, no wonder, I thought. Then a week later, it started getting harder and harder to just ignore the pain or the fact that something was not right. Both my legs started to hurt and my arms sometimes felt numb. And then without any warning, I began to fall over for no reason at all! Now, just imagine walking down the busiest street in your city, a "walking street" where all you can see is a long trail of people going up and down and then you fall down, your body just drops to the ground and you don't know why ... and to make matters even worse you almost fall over 10 more times after that.

And one morning, while you were feeling very proud to say to anybody who would listen that you had 4 kids and yet at 40 years old you still wore a size 0, you realize that you cannot put on that pair of jeans you wore just the week before because now you've gained 10 more centimeters around your waistline. All you can say is "Oh my God, what is happening, this can't be real, what's wrong with me?!" Sitting on your bed, you start sobbing because you don't know what's going on and as if falling over was not already bad enough, now you are bloated like a balloon and you go into panic mode.

Then when you think how on earth can it get any worse, you start dropping everything. You realize that you cannot carry anything anymore because you will probably lose it thanks to gravity. You just have no idea…but life goes on, right? You have the kids, you have your business, you have your world and you need to be strong. You need to put on your poker face regardless because if you show people that you are scared, they'll get frantic and will freak out on you.

At this point I needed some serious answers and I meant it. I could barely walk and my husband had the nerve to tell me that he wanted to buy a wheelchair in a desperate attempt to help me. And no, you don't want to hear what happened to him after that episode!

The first sign of help from the Universe was a chance encounter with John Allen, a chiropractor from New York who had established himself in Sitges, near Barcelona. He is the one who put me back on my two feet and made me walk again. When I think that I almost quit after one session. Yes, because the truth is that it hurt like crazy for 2 days after my 20 minute session with him, as if I were not suffering enough already. But I eventually went back again and again.

This was the physical breakdown I was going through and as if that wasn't enough, my brain started to take momentary vacations as well. I was suffering from serious vertigo, where I would be stuck in my bed for days at a time. And when my brain decided to leave, that's when I finally hit rock bottom. I was aware that my mental faculties were still there, but I couldn't use them, it was all becoming so elusive. What I'm trying to say is that I knew everything I wanted to say, yet the words coming out of my mouth were just gibberish as if I were drunk (even at 6am!). I knew what to do, but my hands and legs had taken on a mind of their own so I couldn't rely on my gestures anymore. I knew what to think, yet my brain was in a thick fog, which made all intellectual tasks impossible to perform even though I was aware of my incapacity. I felt terrible, I felt limited, reduced and so not in control of what was going on. Each time my brain went into "Brain Dead" mode as I got used to calling it, I was going through deeply depressing episodes. At the time, I could have dealt with being physically incapacitated but I certainly was not capable of being intellectually diminished. The thought was unbearable; I couldn't let that happen to me.

This is when we started the never-ending cycle of testing, waiting, nothing; we had to do it all again. Then I got a little breather about 2 weeks before Christmas….I was feeling better. What a wonderful Christmas gift. It's also around this time that we began to understand that I most likely had an Immune Degenerative Disease and, more specifically, Multiple Sclerosis.

That diagnosis was actually liberating. At least I had a label, I knew the 'what' and I had an idea of what doctors wanted me to do to supposedly feel better. However, rather than just counting on them, I would also do my homework. The day I got the neurologist's prescription, I visited my online friend: Google!

That's when I realized that the treatment they had recommended I take did very little to heal the disease and was actually doing a lot to ensure you got even sicker. So I said no way. I told my husband that I refused to kill other organs in my body just to feel as if I'm doing something. I knew there was another way and I was on a mission to find it. And, yes, I did find it.

First of all, I happened to come across a video by Williams Montel, who had gone through the same thing. This video proved to me that it wasn't over, that I could do something about my health and recover some of it. So I embarked on a health mission. My goal was to identify alternative ways to improve my health as fast as I could and in the most meaningful way possible. Among the many things I changed in my life or implemented as new was my diet. I had been a vegetarian all my life (simply because I don't like meat, chicken or fish) so I thought of myself as a pretty healthy woman. But then after reading research papers and articles from various sources I had no choice but to declare that I was not that healthy after all. I was eating A LOT OF pasta, with no meat and with a lot of vegetables, but, nonetheless, pasta. I was eating sandwiches, vegetarian-style and with organic whole wheat, yet still sandwiches and I loved my coffee so much! So I discovered how bad gluten could be for you, I discovered a new world of raw 'un-cooking' and I started experimenting. I remember the first cauliflower couscous I ate, it tasted like the first time I had ever eaten couscous. The flavors were so intense. One meal and I was hooked. Then, yes, I quit pasta—cold turkey (no pun intended). So in one month I became 80% raw and 20% vegan. I still needed the warmth of certain dishes. And I was 150% organic. I started taking a few supplements as well; 50 billion probiotics was number one, then I added vitamin D, vitamin C, vitamin E, L-carnitine, DHA, potassium and magnesium.

I had to admit I was feeling better, so much better that I was able to walk like anyone else. Yes, I was feeling better but that wasn't enough. Simultaneously I worked on a different level; my mindset on one side and my spirituality on the other. So I had created a full protocol for myself targeting my Mind, my Soul and my Body.

THE WORK OF THE BODY

I worked on my body from the inside out, through the food I was consuming. I always made sure it was living and organic ingredients and then as soon as my body allowed, I went back to walking every night, 5 minutes on the treadmill until I could run again for a full 1 hour. Three months after my diagnosis I was at the gym down the street, working out up to 2 hours a day.

It didn't happen like that from one day to the next. It was progressive but every minute mattered to me and every move as well. Along with the chiropractic sessions 3 times a week, I created a program to work on essential motor skills. My program included weights to increase bone density and strength, running and hiking for endurance and Pilates for flexibility. I especially needed to keep my body focused on getting better and I had to give it the right tools; high nutrient foods and the proper way to move. Every move was tailored to work certain muscles in a certain way or in a certain combination. The goal was to re-educate my body to perform everyday moves without any difficulty. A few months later I also hired a personal trainer to bring me back into shape so I could ensure that the next time I was faced with a bad episode, my body would be strong enough to cope with it….or to simply try and avoid the next episode all together.

THE WORK OF THE MIND

I was convinced back then, and I still am today if not more so, that our mind has more power than it would seem at first glance. There are too many accounts of miracles happening every day to simply dismiss them as pure coincidences. I used the following hypothesis; knowing that most of us are raised into thinking negatively about almost everything and especially ourselves and because what we focus on expands, what if I could achieve the same result by brain washing myself into thinking positively? What if I could bring positive things into my life because I spend more time thinking positively rather than negatively?

Thus, my work was set. I started working on my mind almost full-time. I was constantly reading, listening and learning anything I could find. One imposed rule: it had to be uplifting, it had to be positive, and it had to make me feel a better person. Instead of watching TV, I was reading in my bed, and as soon as a doubtful thought crossed my mind I would show it the front door, and wish it good luck with the next mind it found. Then I got my family involved. That wasn't intentional but they liked to try and catch me out as soon as the negative me would rear its ugly head and they would be right there to pounce on it. It actually helped a lot….to make me accountable.

One of the many books I read during that period and which had the most impact on me was The Power of Intention by Wayne Dyer. That book really saved me on the mind level. So much so that it actually helped me leap into the other work I was doing. I also read Breaking the Habit of Being Yourself: How to Lose Your Mind and Create a New One by Dr. Joe Dispenza, The Intention Experiment: Using your Thoughts to Change your Life and the World, by Lynne McTaggart, all the Conversations with God series by Neale Donald Walsch and so many more.

THE WORK OF THE SOUL

I established a strict and disciplined lifestyle for myself. I was up at 4:30am every day, starting my day with a wonderful guided meditation to open up the communication with my Soul. This strategy helped me start each day with clarity which, of course, was fantastic for alleviating brain fog. It also helped me connect with my intuition and then naturally to trust it in my decision-making. In many instances, I was amazed by the synchronicity that was presented to me. I've never felt so vibrant and alive. I had that deep conviction of being in the right place at the right time. For the first time in my life I had a taste of what joy was all about; that deep contented feeling of just being. Mere words fail to describe the feeling I experienced over that period.

I started with a 10 minute meditation. I wanted to feel comfortable in my body first. Being able to stay put without experiencing pain in my legs was a challenge in itself, let alone trying to free my mind from thinking. As time went by and practice continued, I learned to welcome the thoughts, I learned to thank them for stopping by and I learned to say goodbye to them as well. Then the magic materialized! I started missing it if I was late or if I didn't meditate for whatever reason. It became me, it became a way of life. This practice helped me manage my depressive moments a lot better. I had a safe place I could go to whenever I needed or wanted to. The tranquility you get from taking the time to be with yourself and that higher power is precious and nothing else I know provides the same level of peace and quiet.

Alongside my morning meditation, I was also journaling but in a special way. I call it my Gratitude Journal. Every morning I'd light a candle on my desk and I would write down all the things I was grateful for that had happened the day before. I was grateful for the ability to walk. I was grateful for the fantastic weather. I was grateful for the little bird that had visited me the previous morning. I was grateful for many things that I took for granted before I got sick. I was grateful for many things that I knew I wanted to see happening and that I was certain would occur at one point. There is no better way to start your day than by saying Hi to the Universe and to thank it for the wonderful day you know you are going to have.

Today, years later, I'm still persuaded that I couldn't have healed myself so fast if I had not understood the working of these 3 pillars. None of them are any better than the others, none of them are above the others. All of them are required. They work synergistically to ensure homeostasis in our body, in our mind and in our heart.

Each one of us has all we need to feel better....all that matters is to start from where we are and to do it now.

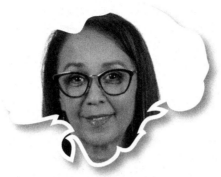

Linda Jenkins

"Feel amazing on the inside—Look amazing on the outside"

Linda is passionate about helping you to look and feel your best from the inside out, and with her range of health and wellness products she has something to offer everyone.

With nearly 40 years working in typical 9-5 work environments, Linda wanted a different way to work, so she set about discovering it. What she discovered was not just a better lifestyle for herself but also a way to use her natural talents and gifts, and make a positive difference in the lives of others.

Linda created her business Amazing Lips to empower other woman to live their best lives, create independent incomes and be the most amazing versions of themselves.

Contact Linda:

28 Tyrrell Rd Jamboree Heights Brisbane Qld Australia, 4074

www.amazinglips.com.au

📞 **+61 413597741**

🅂 **lindilou58891**

f **facebook.com/AmazinglipsAus**

CHAPTER 18

STRENGTH

By Linda Jenkins

I found the strength to pick up a book and keep reading. This simple act changed the course of my health and life.

I had three sons; my eldest son (John) passed away three weeks after being born with a hole in his heart. He would have been 42 years old now.

Two years later, I gave birth to my second son, Lloyd. When he was 14 months old, we moved to Australia. My marriage to my first husband was not a good one as he did not like working and was into drugs. It was two years after we arrived in Australia that my marriage ended. Once again, my life fell apart; I could not understand why I could not have any luck on my side. I went a bit wild during that time; all I wanted was for someone to love me for who I was, but I was going about it the wrong way, which I did not realize until years later.

I met my second husband, Dan, about 12 months after my divorce. At first, things were great, and everybody used to say they wish they had what we had, even though we had our challenges. During the relationship, I was diagnosed with leukemia, and I was raising a young son from my first marriage. We were together for 10 years before we decided to get married, and two years later, I got pregnant with my youngest son, Shane.

We were both so shocked by my pregnancy as neither one of us wanted another child. My eldest son was 14 years old at the time of me falling pregnant, and another child was not what we had planned. Dan and I had a huge fight when we found out I was pregnant with Shane, and that was the beginning of the end of our marriage.

After Shane was born, Danny became so jealous of Shane and the time I spent with him that we started fighting nonstop. At first, the fights were just arguing, and then they started to get physical and then very violent. People often asked me why did I not leave, and I said that when you are so afraid of someone and they have made you feel worthless for so many years, you start to believe what they have been saying. It was the night after a huge fight when Danny had placed a gun to my head that I knew I had to get Shane and myself out of there before he killed me or both of us.

Lloyd was 22 by this stage and had moved out of the house and was working.

He could not live under the same roof as us anymore and watch what Danny was doing to me.

One night in the middle of winter after Danny had fallen asleep, I woke Shane up at 1:00 am, wrapped him in a blanket, and put him in the car. Then, I went back into the house, got my handbag and a change of clothes for the two of us; I got into the car and rolled it down the driveway so that Danny could not hear the car start up. We left and lived at my parents for a short time until I was able to move into a place of my own. I was working and making good money at this stage so that was not a problem. When Danny found out where we were living he started to harass me again, so I moved out of the area to a place that was too far for him to come over all of the time, but close enough for Shane to visit his dad.

Things started to settle down. I had made a lot of friends through work and around the area I was living; one of those people was Francis. He and I had become best mates, nothing else. I only thought of Francis as a friend when I was married to Danny. It was three years after my marriage broke up that Francis and I started dating one another in a more serious way, and we are still together today after 17 years. He taught me to love and respect myself for who and what I was.

Everything was going well. We were all happy. The boys liked Francis because they could see that he treated their mother like a princess.

Then on the 14th of December 2004, my world came tumbling down when I received a call that no parent ever wants to get. Shane, my youngest son, committed suicide at his dad's home; he was 15 years old. Why? I don't know, because out of my two children he was the one that was so happy and full of life. He and I had the most amazing relationship, so for me that was twice as hard to come to terms with. I would not have survived had it not been for Francis and my best friend Chris. It took everything they had to keep me alive. All I did was drink and smoke; I was not eating, sleeping, working, or doing anything.

It took me nine years to start feeling any normality, and I was just starting to think, "God, I am going to make it."

Then Lloyd was killed in a car accident on the 3rd of February 2013; he was 39 years old. I still remember that day like it was yesterday. There was a knock on the door at 1:40 am. I knew before I even answered it that it was bad news, and I remember saying to myself, "I am not going down the same track that I did with Shane with the drinking, smoking, not eating sleeping, or working."

Oh, it ripped my heart apart, but for whatever reason something changed in me at that moment, and I found the strength to stay strong and started thinking of how I was going to turn my life around after losing everything.

I am strong. I had overcome Leukemia, going through all the treatments while raising a young son, followed by the domestic violence in my marriage. The death of my sons, however, was the last straw.

I was sitting in the lounge one evening looking at all my books when it hit me to start reading some of those motivational books I had. So, I went to my library of books and sat on the floor for hours contemplating which book to read. One book kept jumping out at me; it was a book my mum had given me years ago, but until now I could not get into it. I pulled it out and sat on the floor and started reading it.

I am not sure what it was but that book started me reading so many other books. It was called *TNT, The Power within You, How to release the forces inside you and get what you want*, by Claude M. Bristol and Harold Sherman.

And this lead me to Neale Donald Walsh's series of books called *CONVERSATIONS WITH GOD*. Then, *Anatomy of the Spirit, The Seven Stages of Power and Healing*, by Caroline Myss. *The Healer Within* followed that, and then *New Medicine of Mind and Body*, by Steven Locke and Douglas Colligan. I then read *Let Your Feelings Be Your Guide*, by Ester and Jerry Hicks.

It was the start of my journey to turn my life around. Those books and the support of friends taught me how to change my way of thinking about life. It has not been easy, and believe me, I am not out of the woods yet. It has only been two and a half years since Lloyd's passing. Every day I wake up and I thank God for blessing me with everything I have in my life now, the strength to keep going, and the years he gave me with my three sons.

I have made a promise to my sons, to God, but most of all to myself that I will keep myself safe and strong. I have changed quite a lot in my life since losing the boys. I've made changes in the way I think and see things; I now surround myself with positive people.

Twelve months ago, I started my own business called Amazinglips. I sell healthcare products. That has done so much for me in regards to healing myself and giving me the strength to keep going, even though there will always be a void in my life not having my boys with me. They are not here now, but I am, and I still have a lot of people that love me and need me in their lives.

Reading all those books and starting my business and surrounding myself with beautiful, loving, caring, positive people has changed me so much, but it has also shown me that no matter how hard life gets if you change the way you think, if you believe in yourself and respect yourself and surround yourself with positive people, anything is possible.

I have not smoked for 10 years now and drink only in moderation. Since I have been listening to my inner-self and my gut feelings and living for today, things are happening like miracles. My life is what it is meant to be at the moment. I cannot do anything about the past or about tomorrow. For me, it is living in the now and rejoicing in it.

I listened to a message Oprah Winfrey put on her Facebook page. Her words were so powerful, it hit me with such a punch, that I wrote those words down, and I say them to myself every day. What she said is so true, you and you alone can change your life around, nobody else. This is what she said:

"You are responsible for your life and if you sit around waiting for someone to save you, fix you, or help you, you're wasting your time because only you have the power to take responsibility to move your life forward."

What matters is now, this moment, and your willingness to see this moment for what it is, accept the past, take responsibility, and move forward.

I came to realize that I was praying for God to do something, and God was waiting for me to do something. How true is this? We are all guilty of this, but God will help us once we look within ourselves.

So start today and change your life, for you have the power within you to do that. And remember you have the strength to do it.

I would like to share this with all of you. My son Shane used to write poetry, and this is one of his poems, printed here exactly the way he wrote it.

TO MUM

A poem 4 u
When you are sad
I will dry your tears
When you are scared
I will comfort your fears
When you are worried
I will give you hope
When you are confused
I will help u cope
And when you are lost
And can't find the light
I shall be your beacon
Shining ever so bright
This is my oath I pledge till the end
Why you ask?
Because you are my mum

By Shane Jenkins

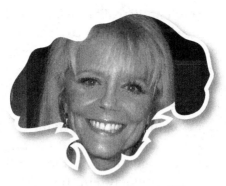

Sunny Griffin

A BEAUTIFUL LIFE

For Sunny Griffin, looking and feeling great is not just a career move, it's a way of life. In 1966 she was the world's highest-paid Supermodel. Today, at age 74, she is a leading beauty and fitness expert. Her self-described mission in life is to help people reach their own personal fitness and beauty goals. Sunny spent two and-a-half years as the health and beauty correspondent for ABC's Good Morning America and has continued to make television and personal appearances throughout the country, establishing a loyal following as a health and beauty motivational "guru."

Sunny's face and figure appeared regularly throughout the '60s and '70s on national and international magazine covers. She was also featured in literally hundreds of television commercials. Throughout this time she appeared in several off-Broadway productions and, in 1969, landed a plum role opposite Dustin Hoffman in the film "John and Mary".

Sunny's longtime interest and expertise in beauty and fashion along with her vivacious personality and positive outlook on life soon led her to pursue a second career as a motivational speaker, helping people improve their lives and self-esteem through exercise, better nutrition and positive thinking.

In 1994, Sunny and her family realized a lifelong dream and moved to Telluride, Colorado, where she decided to tie her interests in health, beauty, cosmetics, fashion and business together and founded her own company, SunStar Dimensions. In the summer of 1997, SunStar introduced a revolutionary new line of raw botanical skincare products, "Astara Skin Care." By utilizing a unique anti-oxidizing skincare technology combined with living botanical ingredients Sunny's line of Astara Skin Care products harnesses the power of nature to effect real changes in skin tone, anti-aging and overall health. Today, Sunny's uniquely effective Astara product line has become an astonishing success in spas and specialty stores across the USA as well as numerous resorts and boutiques all over the world.

Contact Sunny

www.astaraskincare.com

 facebook.com/astaraskincare

CHAPTER 19

LIVING RAW

By Sunny Griffin

I learned very early on how important a healthy lifestyle is. For me, it was a job requirement since a model must be thin and have good skin. I do not come from a family of thin people. In fact, it is quite the opposite, and I am sure I never once heard the word nutrition mentioned when growing up. I remember an argument I had with my mother when I started my skin care company and created botanical products that were free of chemicals. My mother insisted "chemicals are good for you," a phrase I assume she learned from DuPont ads in the 1950s.

I was very lucky because my career forced me to learn everything possible to keep my body thin and fit and as healthy as possible. Modeling is not a career that allows sick days, and a top model works so much there is no time to eat. So I carried sliced carrots, celery, zucchini, red pepper, apples, pears, etc. in my model-bag so I would have something nutritious to eat and have energy without gaining weight. It turns out that I was a raw foodist even in the 1960s before I had ever heard of the concept of raw food. At that time, the primary advantage was that it was portable and it kept me nourished and healthy. Eating a very healthy diet from my early 20s is possibly why most junk food doesn't even appeal to me, because my body recognizes that it is not good for me.

Fast forward to 1994. I am still living an extremely healthy lifestyle. I am 54 and speaking in front of a room of about 200 people when my entire left side goes numb. It was a TIA (mini-stroke) and only lasted a few minutes, but I had two more TIAs over the next two days. I rushed to the doctor who told me my left carotid artery was 95% blocked. WHAT??? How can this happen to a health nut like me? Emergency surgery that day was an incision the entire length of my neck to clean out the plaque built up in the artery and left me with a raised scar that frightened people for years. This sort of thing happens to people who lead a sedentary life, eat poorly, and smoke... the absolute opposite of me. But everyone on both sides of my family had died either from strokes, heart attacks, or hardening of the arteries. I have genetic vascular disease, and there is nothing I can do about it according to my doctors. After my first carotid artery surgery, I was told it would be 6 to 12 weeks before I recovered. I was back at work in two weeks, the result of being very healthy before surgery. Ten years later, my right carotid artery dissected intra-cranially (meaning it became damaged in my head), and I had my first brain surgery. I have now had seven brain surgeries and have recovered easily from every one and have been told over and over by every doctor I have seen that my lifestyle is why I heal so well.... if only a healthy lifestyle could correct my genetic vascular disease. I now have stents in two carotid arteries in my head and coils in two aneurysms in my brain.

At 69 years old, I was in a very serious auto accident in Thailand. The driver was a 23 year old girl, and we were on an open highway when a dog ran in front of the car. She swerved to avoid hitting the dog, and the car crashed into a concrete power pole at 68 km per hour. The front of the car was crushed in like an accordion. We were both wearing seat belts, but the air bags did not go off. My back was broken in three places, a disc in the middle of my back was crushed, and my neck was pulverized. The girl who was driving only got serious whiplash, which shows you how much more brittle bones get as we age. The doctors in the hospital kept saying (in their Thai accent) it was "unbereaveable" that I survived. I was told that my neck was so crushed that it was too dangerous to do surgery, and I was put in a metal brace to completely immobilize my neck. I was not allowed to fly for five weeks, and my daughter had to fly to Thailand to accompany me back to the USA in a wheelchair.

I saw the leading neck surgeon in the USA who said my neck could be fixed, but he could not operate until the crushed bones had time to solidify and that would take three months. I was put in a brace that went from my hips to the top of my head and screwed in place.

There would be no hair washing or bathing, other than sponge baths, for the next six months. The metal brace was miserable and made it almost impossible to sleep. After three months, I had spinal surgery to put two titanium rods, five screws, and what they said was a "pulley system" (but looks kind of like a paper clip in the X-ray) in my neck. I was told I had to be back in that brace for a minimum of six months, but probably more because of my age.

That is when I decided to eat only 100% raw organic food with all the enzymes active to help my body heal itself. To the astonishment of the doctors, I was out of the brace and into physical therapy after two months and three weeks rather than the more than six months they had predicted.

What is it about raw food that has such seemingly magical qualities? It is that the enzymes are still active. Enzymes are the spark of life. Nothing happens without them. We couldn't move a muscle or have a thought without enzymes. But enzymes cannot survive heat. At 105°Fahrenheit (40.5°C) they begin to be destroyed, and at 118°F (48°C) they are completely denatured, unable to do anything in our bodies.

There is so much confusion today about what is the healthiest kind of diet, and I strongly believe we should focus as much as possible on eating organic foods in their natural raw state because they contain all the essential components our bodies need, in the form we need them. Raw food helps to alkalize the body, which we now know is the key to building excellent health. When the body is in an alkaline state it can absorb nutrients and expel toxins much better The Standard American Diet (with the delightful acronym: SAD) consisting of meat, bread, dairy products, processed/cooked foods, caffeine, and alcohol creates an acidic state in the body that can contribute to all kinds of health problems.

Every raw whole food contains enzymes designed by nature to break down that particular food so our bodies don't have to use up the enzymes we make to digest food, and those enzymes are available to produce the energy we need to fuel our cells and their many activities. Enzymes are the labor force of the body and are involved in every single process of our bodies. But since they cannot survive heat, they are completely destroyed in any food that has been canned, Pasteurized, baked, roasted, stewed, or fried. Processing, refining, cooking, and microwaving denatures all the enzymes and causes imbalances and stress on our organs and body tissue which causes cellular exhaustion and can lay the foundation for a weak immune system and decrease the longevity of the body. This becomes much more important as we age because the body loses its ability to manufacture enzymes. Young adults have 30 times the enzymes of the elderly. When you think of it, age is not so much the number of years you have lived, but the integrity of your body tissues. Our goal for optimum health and longevity should be to conserve our body's enzymes for use in repairing and rebuilding rather than deplete them in digestion.

Cooked and processed foods (which 95% of people eat 95% of the time) have no healing power what-so-ever, which is why most doctors don't understand that food can heal. Yet Hippocrates, the Father of Modern Medicine, said 2000 years ago: "Let food be thy medicine and medicine be thy food." People are healed from many diseases by changing to a raw food diet, but wouldn't you rather prevent a problem rather than having to cure it? Our bodies are miraculous, self-healing machines if given the right fuel. 90%, or more, of cardiovascular disease can be cured by lifestyle choices. 60%, or more of cancers can be cured by lifestyle choices. The American Diabetes Association says: "Diabetes is a chronic disease that has no cure," yet Gabriel Cousens cures diabetes in 30 days on a raw food diet at his "Tree of Life Rejuvenation Center" in Patagonia, Arizona. Gabriel says: "Genetics loads the gun; Lifestyle pulls the trigger."

The USA has the most overweight population in the history of humanity! We have more hospitals, more medicines, more doctors than ever before, and we are getting sicker. We need the micro-nutrients that are only in raw food. When you cook food, you lose 50% of the protein, 70—85% of the vitamins and minerals, and 100% of the phyto-nutrients. And believe me, nothing tastes as good as the feeling of being fit and having energy.

It is not necessary to eat 100% raw food to be healthy. My goal is 70 to 80% raw (unless I am in a healing crisis when I eat 100% raw), and I suggest you start small and take it a step at a time. I have found the concept of "I can't have this and I can't have that" leads to feelings of deprivation so it is easier to add raw dishes to your diet and slowly eliminate less healthy ones as you replace them with the thousands of delightful raw options out there. Today there are hundreds of raw cook books on the market and limitless raw recipes on the internet. Simply google what you like. For example, if you like Shepherd's Pie google "Raw Shepherd's Pie" for a wonderful raw recipe. My husband loves mashed potatoes and gravy so I make it using raw cauliflower and mushrooms. I make lemon cheesecake from cashew nuts, and no one can believe it has no cheese. I also make the most amazing "Chocolate of the Gods" from avocados and raw cacao. Chips and guacamole are wonderful when the chips are made from real corn and dehydrated at a low temperature. There is a world of wonderful raw food out there waiting to take you to a life of radiant good health. I am 75 years old and now feel secure in telling you: Raw Food works!

CHAPTER 20

MY STORY IS ABOUT THAT

By Anna Suvorova

When asked by a beautiful co-author of *One Crazy Broccoli* to share my self-healing story, I had to pause and reflect on what was it that I really wanted to say. There are so many ways to tell our stories, so many ways to share what is in our hearts. At the end of the day, it all comes to what we have chosen to believe.

On one hand, I am a person living with an auto-immune disorder. I am not taking any pharmaceuticals and am making a tremendous effort to live as conscious and natural as is possible in our modern plastic-fantastic world. Dealing with the side effects of medical drugs seems as scary to me as dealing with the illness itself. My life feels like a constant battle between opposite forces: health and sickness, vitality and exhaustion. Being unaware is a luxury I cannot afford. It might cost me my life. I have to watch every step I take and every choice I make: what foods go into my body, what emotions I allow, and what energies I engage in. Being sick has showed me how fragile and vulnerable we actually are, how interconnected everything is.

On the other hand, I am this person who has chosen to step out of the ordinary to find my own truth. I feel like with this challenge of being sick I was invited to expand and break free from my own limitations. I find myself being on the most exciting journey of non-stop discovering of new ways of being a human being. I search and learn, and I never stop experimenting on myself. I have experienced numerous diets, detoxes, and healing techniques. I have read the most extraordinary books written by remarkable human beings who traveled to the mystery zone, a place that is outside of the ordinary and accepted norm. Thanks to being unwell, I have tapped into the knowledge I would have never known about. Thanks to it, I have learned that there are no limits to how far we can expand.

We have been programed to live within the box; our limitations have been accepted as the norm. I see my story being about breaking out of that box, it is about changing our beliefs and daring to reprogram who we are and who we choose to be.

It has been a privilege to have a physical challenge. I live in a super sensitive human body that reacts to anything unnatural: food, light, environment, etc. Since a very young age, my body has experienced a lot of pain, and that is how it became my greatest teacher. When our body is unwell, we cannot do much apart from being still and present to what IS. And when we become that, we can tap into the deeper truth of this sensational experience—being a human being.

I have lived with what is called lupus since I was 14, my state of health was confusing me and all those around me all the way until I was finally diagnosed with it at 31. At first I cried, feeling sorry for myself, then I raged at the fact of how unfair life was, and then, finally, I accepted the challenge. This invitation to grow and to find my truth has become my life. When I refused to take medications, I did not really know what I was doing, I just knew what I wanted to believe. I chose to believe that by eating healthy, staying clean, and making choices that served my higher good I would heal. What did I do? Everything. I totally changed the way I lived…

Sometimes we have to die before we start living, and that is what changing myself felt like. I packed up my life in a big polluted city (in London), gave everything away, and moved closer to nature, to a small island (in Thailand) where I was taking beach walks and watching the stars, learning Reiki and yoga, and just being happy. I connected with many others who were on similar journeys, and there was comfort in that. I had to transform from a person I knew how to be into someone I never thought I could be or expected to be. I came to see that there is no healing without transformation.

As I look back at this long exciting journey that I have embarked upon, I do not really wish to talk about how I traveled to India to live in an ashram and took long pilgrimages or how many times I fasted and gazed at the sun. I do not wish to discuss those long hours spent on the yoga mat just breathing and learning to be whatever I have been. There is no point talking about the silent retreats or mind-altering meditation and chanting. Those are just the tools. What I do wish to say is this—Nothing changes until we do. There is no healing without transformation, without willingness to change and rearrange everything we have learned and accepted about ourselves. At the end of the day, it all comes to what we have chosen to believe. My story is about that.

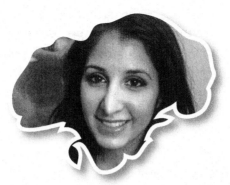

Dr. Maral Yazdandoost

Dr. Maral is a Canadian naturopathic doctor specializing in pain management and injury recovery. She has additional certification in Applied Kinesiology, Mesotherapy and Biopuncture, as well as Facial Rejuvenation Acupuncture (cosmetic acupuncture). She is a graduate of the Canadian College of Naturopathic Medicine and holds an Honours Bachelor of Science from McMaster University, specializing in Biology and Psychology.

Believing strongly in the interconnection of body, mind and spirit, Dr. Maral was drawn to alternative medicine at an early age. In discovering Naturopathic Medicine, she knew she had found a discipline which emphasized this interconnection and satisfied her passion for understanding the human body with its structural, biochemical and emotional interplay.

The diverse scope of Naturopathic Medicine allows Dr. Maral to individualize comprehensive treatment to fully address all aspects of presenting conditions, while taking into account her patients unique requirements. Dr. Maral makes ample use of acupuncture, nutritional supplements and botanical formulations. She is also a compassionate counsellor and understands the inherent wisdom of a clean diet, physical therapies and preventative medicine.

She offers safe, natural, integrative therapies for many commonly presenting conditions. She is also a compassionate advocate for mental health and stress management focusing on treating anxiety and depression without pharmaceutical drugs. Above all, she is passionate about educating and empowering patients to optimize their health. She is available for private consultation and for corporate wellness programs and encourages you to take charge of your health, today!

Contact Dr. Maral:

www.DrMaral.com

✉ **dr.maral.nd@gmail.com**

f **facebook.com/Dr.Maral.ND**

@DrMaralND

@Dr_Maral

CHAPTER 21

FEAR NOT! HOW TO BREAK THROUGH THE STIGMA AND MASK OF ANXIETY DISORDER

By Dr. Maral Yazdandoost, ND

As a naturopathic doctor, my patients often ask me what it was that first drew me to this form of medicine instead of the conventional medical model. Since a large portion of my practice is focused on acute and chronic pain management, most patients are surprised to hear that I initially entered the field to explore and share natural, non-pharmaceutical treatments for mental health disorders.

I credit my own personal experiences in dealing with anxiety as the reason I ultimately turned away from conventional medicine in favor of pursuing a more holistic, integrative system of health. It began in my last year of high school, though I'm sure I had perfectionistic tendencies and an unhealthy relationship with control long before that. Certain classes, certain exams, and even certain social circumstances with my peers would cause my heart to sink, before beating wildly. Then it would become harder to breathe, my lungs never seeming to get enough oxygen no matter how much or how deeply I breathed. Though I knew something was wrong, it was all too vague, too difficult to describe, so I didn't tell anyone. Initially, I shrugged it all off as random, isolated events.

When I graduated high school and left to attend university in another city, I wasn't thinking of these vague episodes. I was excited to start a new chapter of my life, to live on my own, and meet new people. I saw the next four years as preparation for medical school, and I had no time for anxiety. Yet somehow, anxiety managed to find me. And slowly, over the first few months of university, my anxiety deepened.

What had started as random, isolated events intensified and started happening more frequently. I began to experience them a few times per week. At the same time, I realized that I was also gaining weight. A lot of it. I felt hungry all the time and was gaining weight despite being more active than before. And new symptoms emerged: an internal trembling that would crescendo to violent shaking and a feeling of dread that grew into outright fear. The fear was insidious and pervasive, and because I never knew exactly what it was I was afraid of, I felt as if I was stalked by my own fear.

Yet, I still didn't tell anyone about these events precisely because they seemed so unusual, so abnormal. After all, I was a straight-A student, had a great group of friends, and was planning on studying medicine. What would people think if they knew of these symptoms? How would they judge me? They would probably just tell me it was all in my head.

Things finally came to a head when I had a severe episode while watching a movie with a friend at our dorm room. I was now in my second year of university, and my anxiety was an open secret among my tight circle of friends. Almost all my friends had seen me struggle to breathe, while trembling too violently to remain standing. Some had even had to escort me to class, because my nameless terror made it difficult to leave my room. They were concerned, but I kept shrugging it off. On this particular night, my friend said that I looked like I was having convulsions and could not speak. She called the campus emergency services as I blacked out. When they arrived, they had to administer oxygen to revive me. Looking at the group of first responders, my friends, and all the others who had come to investigate, I knew that this situation was no longer just in my head. It was out of my control.

In the days that followed, I finally admitted to myself that something was wrong and set about to find out what it was. I was studying Biology and Psychology, because I had always had a strong interest in the connection between the mind and the body. I drew on this academic background to quickly identify my acute symptoms as descriptive of panic attacks. Taking into account the nameless fears and anxieties I experienced almost daily, I determined that I must be suffering from Panic Disorder. Armed with this knowledge, I made an appointment at my campus health center. I wanted to ask my medical doctor to give me a referral for cognitive behavioral therapy. My doctor, however, was reluctant. As she explained it, any anxiety I was feeling was likely circumstantial due to the stress of school. "After all," she asked, "do you really want a psychiatric evaluation on your permanent medical record?"

This was the first time that I experienced the stigmatization of mental health disorders, as well as the complacency of the conventional medical system. My doctor never explored any of my fears and did not order any blood work for me. She simply sent me away with a sample pack of antidepressants and a vague recommendation to "cut back on caffeine." I was crushed. Having suffered silently with these panic attacks for over three years before finally admitting I needed help, it was demoralizing to be dismissed so quickly. I didn't even drink coffee.

Yet I could no longer continue to suffer. I did not want to take antidepressants that I knew could cause more weight gain, so I quit drinking black tea and continued searching for answers. I still had panic attacks, so there had to be something that I was missing. Something that could give me back a sense of control. One afternoon as I sat at my computer doing research for a psychology assignment, I found that certain something. I stumbled upon a list of symptoms that sounded eerily familiar: elevated heart rate, shortness of breath, unexplained fear, and violent trembling or shaking. Losing consciousness was listed as the most severe symptom if left untreated. The diagnosis: *hypoglycemia.* Low blood sugar.

This seemingly simple concept would become a liberating force for me. My background in biology, having been pushed aside by my own insistence that this was "all in my head," i.e. psychological, now came rushing back to connect the dots for me. A reliable pattern finally emerged. I had a strong family history of diabetes and had struggled with weight gain, and most importantly, I had noticed that certain meals increased my anxiety. I intuitively avoided meals that were heavy in carbohydrates, like pasta or rice, because within twenty minutes of eating them I felt unwell. In my eagerness to establish the connection of the mind to the body, I labeled myself as having a panic disorder, and I ignored the connection the *body* has to the *mind.* My body was suffering and speaking to me in the only language it knew, through my mind and its interpretation of internal and external stimuli.

For the first time in a long while, I felt as if there was hope: if I could learn to control my blood sugar, then the hypoglycemia would stabilize, and my anxiety with it. I was excited to learn more and I threw myself into research, using university resources and my well-honed academic skills.

The term "blood sugar" refers to the level of glucose found in the blood. Glucose is the ultimate breakdown product of most foods containing carbohydrates and it is the body's preferred source of energy. For glucose to enter individual cells of the body, we need a hormone called insulin, which is produced by the pancreas. Insulin is like the key that unlocks the door for glucose to get inside the cells.

For most people, controlling their blood sugar does not require active monitoring or preventative measures. But for people like me, the reaction to carbohydrate-rich foods produces unstable blood sugar levels, often resulting in hypoglycemia. This is due to a number of complex and often interconnected factors including abnormal insulin production, excess stress hormones, and an under functioning thyroid gland or inflammation. Whatever the reason, the end result is the same—most susceptible people experience a host of symptoms including anxiety, mental confusion, trouble concentrating, and light-headedness. I had experienced all these symptoms and more, which is why I was so motivated to learn how to prevent them.

I started with the most obvious factor: the foods that I was eating. For people who have trouble controlling their blood sugar, meals that are high in carbohydrates should be avoided. In fact, it is best to combine carbohydrates, which are easily digested, with other foods that take longer to digest like proteins or fat. I began tracking my meals and realized that if I included about 20-25 grams of protein with each meal, I could stabilize my blood sugar much more effectively. For those of you who are wondering, that's roughly one chicken breast or one cup of cooked lentils.

Being a busy student, I quickly realized that there would be days that three large meals would not be practical for me. Eating five to six smaller, nutrient dense meals or snacks actually kept my blood sugar more stable. My favorite snack was a handful of trail mix containing nuts, seeds, and dried fruit. This combination had moderate amounts of protein a good dose of healthy fats, and fiber to keep me going.

My research led me to explore how stress affects the body. When the body is stressed, it shuts down its digestive processes to conserve all its energy for fighting the source of stress. In our modern lives, the sources of stress are not always easy to identify or to remove, which means that hormones like cortisol and adrenaline can be elevated. Chronic elevation of these hormones impairs our glucose response and can lead to worsened hypoglycemia. I reconnected with my practice of meditation to help lower my stress levels and allow me to recharge more effectively. I also began exercising more regularly to promote better elimination of excess hormones from the body.

I felt better than I had in years. The changes in my diet and increased exercise had the added effect of helping me lose weight, and my confidence began to return. I still had panic attacks, but instead of two to three per week, I would have just one per month. It was a definite improvement, but the underlying reasons for my hypoglycemia were still there. By this time I was in my final year of university, and though I had always wanted to study medicine, conventional medicine no longer attracted me. I wanted to practice medicine in an integrative, holistic way, focusing on diet and lifestyle changes to address what I saw as commonly misdiagnosed chronic conditions. Lucky for me, I discovered naturopathic medicine with its focus on the integration of mind, body, and spirit, and its emphasis on treating the whole person, not just the symptoms of disease.

It wasn't until I entered naturopathic medical school that I was able to put the last pieces of my treatment into place. In the course of my studies, I learned that chromium, an element that helps stabilize blood sugar, is often deficient in the North American diet, so I started taking 200 µg per day. I also learned how important the B vitamins are in generating energy within our cells. More importantly, the active forms of vitamin B3 (niacinamide) and vitamin B5 (pantothenic acid) are very important for helping to stabilize anxiety, which is why I still take a high-quality B complex supplement daily.

With this regiment in place, I completely stopped having panic attacks. Of course a certain amount of anxiety is normal and perfectly acceptable in high-stress situations, but I was able to recognize these episodes for what they are. I no longer felt ruled by my fears. I felt back in control. I felt empowered. It is this sense of empowerment that I try to foster in all my patients.

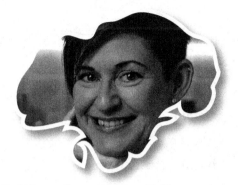

Nicole van Hattem

HHC/AADP, AFAIM, CAHRI

Nicole van Hattem is an international best selling author, wellness guru, Holistic Success Coach, and Host of Hot & Healthy podcast series.

Combining over two decades of corporate experience, with board certification as a holistic health coach, skills as a Master NLP practitioner and a wealth of practical life experience, Nicole skillfully reaches her audience and transforms lives.

A regular guest expert speaker at major cancer awareness events, corporate workshops and community health awareness programs with attendance reaching into the tens of thousands, Nicole is considered a trusted expert in the field of health and wellness.

Nicole's holistic success coaching service is available to those who are serious about their health and taking control of their financial future. As a six-figure business mentor, she ignites the spark in ordinary people and works with them so they can achieve extraordinary healthy wealthy lives.

Contact Nicole:

Website: www.NicolevanHattem.com

✉ nicole@nicolevanhattem.com

f Nicole van Hattem—Success Coach

🐦 @NicolevanHattem

📷 Nicole_van_Hattem

in linked.com/in/nicolevanhattem

CHAPTER 22

FAT, SICK, AND SUCCESSFUL

By Nicole van Hattem

As I sit here in the cancer hospital waiting room drafting my book chapter, I look around at the faces of the other patients and quietly give thanks.

Today is a day to celebrate.

Yes I'm celebrating. Right here in the cancer ward.

I am not here for my own cancer treatment. I'm here to support my mum as she faces terminal cancer. A cancer diagnosis is a terrible reality and a terminal cancer prognosis is nothing short of devastating, regardless of who it is happening to. But I'm being honest. I am grateful that it isn't me who is waiting to discuss my medical treatment with the Oncology Team.

It could just as easily be me. Just a few years ago, I was eating processed junk food at every meal, technically obese and about as active as a caged sloth. Statistically I had lead myself into a high-risk category for any one of the more common chronic diseases, such as diabetes, heart disease, and various types of cancer. I was living a lifestyle that was playing Russian roulette with my health.

And I'd been living this way for decades. I had abused my one precious body from many angles: poor work and lifestyle habits, damaging personal relationships, poor food choices, over the counter medications, and alcohol. When I was in my late thirties and living a high-intensity corporate life, I thought that I would have time to change my lifestyle once I had made it to the top. That I could recover later from the sacrifices I was making with my health now.

I exchanged my health for more time behind my desk, in front of my computer, ticking off lists, stressing more about achieving organizational recognition and gaining financial rewards.

I traded my health for cash. Was it worth it? At the time, yes! In hindsight, what the hell was I thinking? Some part of me at the time knew that I was walking a fine line of good health versus ill health. There had been some hints that my poor lifestyle could eventually rob me of my greatest wealth, my health, but I chose to ignore them. I was afraid to make changes to how I was living my life because it seemed to be working fine as it was. After all I was successful, wasn't I?

Success is a personal definition. I had unconsciously defined success as being able to earn large sums of money, achieve awards, buy luxury items, and go on expensive holidays. Health and wellbeing was the price I was prepared to pay to have these things. At least for a while. I banked on the idea that I would be able to use my money later in my life to recover my looks or even my health if I really needed to. I could pay for surgeries, pills, treatments, and it would all be ok. Wouldn't it?

Surely I would know when enough personal sacrifice was enough, and then I would easily know when I had climbed high enough up the corporate ladder. I would be able to recognize when I was close to my health tipping point and easily make the effort to eat better, sleep better, breath more, move more. The problem was that I had conditioned myself to accept that the discomfort I was feeling in my mind and body as normal, and because I enjoyed the materialistic benefits of the life I had created, I wasn't willing to listen to my body's calls for attention.

My body was putting up little warning flags every day. I efficiently ignored them. Each time my body sent out a message that something was out of balance, I swiftly took action to delete the message. Blurry vision—got my eyes checked and new glasses prescribed. Bleeding gums, aching teeth, cavities—off to the dentist for more fillings, mouthwash, and a toothpaste for sensitive teeth. Headaches, backache, leg-ache—swallowed a painkiller. Erratic heartbeat, anxiety, and panic attacks—blamed on deadlines, office politics, lack of self-confidence, too short holidays, and a husband who just didn't understand me. Weight gain and food addictions—restrictive diets, personal trainers, and bigger clothes. Bloating, gas, heartburn, diarrhea, and constipation—brushed off as normal. Night sweats, painful periods, insomnia, mind fog, hair loss, exhaustion, anger, and depression—I addressed with over the counter medications, caffeine, alcohol, sugary and processed foods.

At 38 years old, the doctors told me that my long list of aches and pains were nothing more than a normal part of ageing and deterioration. So I kept spending my precious time and money covering up my symptoms. But my body loves me and it just didn't give up trying. Eventually, it got my attention. I looked in the mirror and finally realized that I was the cause and the cure of my pain. It was time to wake up and answer my body's symptomatic calls before I received the siren screams of disease.

My initial response to my wakeup call was to go on a detox retreat in Thailand. A raw, vegan bootcamp style detox retreat, where we got up at dawn and walked for 45 minutes in the steamy jungle heat, learned yoga and meditation, juice fasted all day, did coffee colonics (enemas), and were sleeping by 9 pm in a sparse hut. Wow, now that really woke me up. Without the distractions of my normal life, at the retreat I could really listen to my inner wisdom. It was then that I was able to understand how truly sick I was and how close I had taken myself to my tipping point.

After three weeks at the retreat, I returned to my corporate life with a very different perspective on life and a determination to be grateful for my symptoms. To use them as guide posts on my healing journey and in creating the right living style for me. I began to study holistic health and trained as a health coach. Even though I had the commitment to make healthy changes, I had practiced my bad old habits for a very long time, and I was really good at them. My habits had also been providing me with ways with which to cope with my hectic life. It has been six years since then, and the road has been bumpy but the destination is oh-so-worth it.

In the years that have passed, as a result of some simple and sustainable changes I have made in my life, most of my symptoms (warning lights) have been switched off. Instead of moving closer to my tipping point, I have tipped the scale in my favor. "Analysis of global research shows that about a third of the most common cancers are preventable through a nutritious diet, maintaining a healthy weight and regular physical activity.[1]" I eat a highly nutritious wholefoods diet including superfoods such as aloe vera, raw cacao, spirulina, and high quality supplements. I've lost 17 kg of toxic fat off my body and from around my internal organs. I exercise every day and include dancing, yoga, and walking in nature.

When symptoms appear in my own body (my body is smarter than I am), I respond quickly and in sustainable and self-supporting ways. Aches and pains, breathing irregularities, headaches, sleeplessness, and stress still happen from time to time. Now I choose to manage them with breathing exercises, power naps, yoga, meditation, massage, herbal baths, having a good laugh, and surrounding myself with people who nourish me at an emotional level.

I take care of my digestive system every day with aloe vera gel drinks, probiotics, fermented foods, bee propolis, lots of vegetables, generous portions of raw foods, and a little high quality animal products, bowel massage, and rest. Taking care of my digestive system in this way has boosted my immune system, and I rarely suffer with a cold and the flu. When I'm emotional (like I am now, as the primary carer for my mum) or my period is due, I will still choose to eat some processed packaged foods, reach for a few favorite junk foods, eat chocolate and red wine every day, but now I choose the highest qualities I can access and consume much less quantity.

In addition to changing my food style, moving my body more, and managing my stress differently, I also redefined my definition of success and I changed my career path. I believe this has made the most difference in my health and how I contribute to the world. I still have a high intensity work life, but now it is as a Holistic Success Coach guiding others how to listen when their body talks, define

---

[1] World Cancer Research Fund International **www.wcrf.org**

what success means to them, and create vitality and sustainable success in their lives.

So yes, I am celebrating. I have so much to be grateful for, even at this difficult time. I am grateful for the small changes I have made to how I live my life and how this has resulted in a deeper connection with my body's wisdom, an abundance of health, and time to write my story so far.

CHAPTER 23

ACCEPTING DISCOMFORT— DISCOVERING PEACE

Jacki Woodworth

By the time I was 39 years old, I was married with two small children, three part-time jobs, and a raging out of control eating disorder. I didn't understand it at the time but what I have learned since is that I am a compulsive overeater and sugar addict who was tipping the scales at over 280 lbs. To top it off, I had quit smoking when pregnant, but desperate to reduce my weight, I secretly took it up again when my children were little. A desperate desire to control all aspects of my life led me to add compulsive exercise to the list as well. Basically, anything that could keep me numb to the bitter reality that I was unhappy with myself and what I had become.

I grew up on a farm where butter, cream, sugar, and homemade sweets were staples. Love was doled out in hugs, kindness, apple pie, ice cream, and molasses cookies. I was generally a happy child who loved her food! I don't recall ever having an "off" switch. The sugary treats were abundantly available, and no one ever said no. By the time I was ten years old, I was into the husky size jeans and became sadly accustomed to being referred to as a "big girl." As I grew taller (to 180 cm), so I grew in girth. Increasingly self-conscious and ashamed of my size, I soon became a "heavy set" teenager, who ate to numb discomfort, shame, sadness, and, ultimately, anger. I didn't understand the cycle that was developing, all I knew was that I was fat and miserable, and I covered it up with humor and eating more. The more miserable I felt, the more I ate. I found food soothing, and I had a lot to be soothed and no other skills to quiet the growing discontent within. Eating was a coping mechanism that helped me deal with life. Although it was destructive, I could not see another way. A mentor once told me, "People do the best they can with what they know at the time." All I knew about it at that time was that eating seemed to relieve my pain.

At 13, I started my first diet. This began a rollercoaster of weight controlling behaviors that evolved into a disordered, addicted relationship with food and body image. It began with fasting, calorie counting, and compulsive exercise and evolved over 30 years to include binging, purging, dishonesty, and denial—the fundamentals of addictive behavior and misery.

In 2003, we moved to Doha, Qatar. Unbeknownst to me, this was a move that would wake me up—body, mind, heart, and soul. Looking back now, I see that my approach to health began to change as other distractions reduced. Other than my family, I knew no one in Qatar. I was also without work for the first time since I was 12. This is the typical recipe for disaster for an addict, but this time something was different. Instead of running from discomfort, I began to get curious about it. Because my busy life briefly slowed, I began to hear an internal whisper, distant and yet familiar, reminiscent of the one Mary Oliver describes in her poem *The Journey*, "…and there was a new voice which you slowly recognized as your own, that kept you company as you strode deeper and deeper into the world…" As I began to give space to this voice, I began to discover a "me" that had been buried beneath layers of self-deprecation and struggles. I began to "come home" to myself, to the one who could thrive if I listened, nurtured, and allowed her. I explored this "awakening" very slowly on my own for three years during which time I quit smoking, drank more water, and began developing a healthier approach to food and exercise. I lost 20 lbs and plateaued there.

In early 2007, I went back to see a physician I had been pestering about knee pain. She had patiently referred me for everything from x-rays and medication to massage and physio. On this particular visit, she finally said, "Quite frankly, my dear, if you don't do something about your weight your knee will not get better, it will get worse." I was stunned and angry. How dare she?! It took about three days for her wisdom to penetrate the wall of denial. I had just turned 43.

A few weeks later, I found my way to a 12 Step meeting of Overeaters Anonymous. As I sat in that meeting, it was the first time in my life I heard people speak a language around food and eating that I understood. They spoke openly about the twisted and tormented ways they related to food. I had never heard such honesty about something so deeply familiar to me. They spoke of taboo things no one I knew talked about. I felt I had come home — these people were my kin, my tribe! I wept through most of the meeting and began working the 12 steps that day.

The first step requires an admission of powerlessness over food. As a student of feminism, admitting powerlessness about anything was not likely, and yet, as I struggled with it, the truth became clear. I had fought the battle all my life and here I was at 43 — fat, unhealthy, unhappy, and really tired of trying things that never lasted. Clearly, I was powerless, and another diet or more exercise was never going to be the answer.

I took the first small step, I let go of control just for a moment and accepted life as it was. This moment turned into another moment and another, all opportunities to explore this strangeness called acceptance. This way of relating to life has turned into a chain of moments of letting go and accepting. To this day, this practice is the strongest act I commit, and I do so daily. I continue to accept that being human means I'm beautifully and uniquely imperfect and powerless over the twists and turns of life. It means I trust that I have many deep (and often untapped) capacities to meet what life has in store, the ups AND downs. Today I cope without turning to food to numb discomfort. Every day since, today included, I wake up and say thank you to a source much greater and wiser than me and ask, "What's my role here today?" And so it goes, one day at a time — one breath at a time.

In 2007 I also discovered Yoga. I added it to my exercise routine and thought all was good. By 2009, I was in a nine month Yoga teacher training and had discovered mindfulness. This has been the crown of it all for me. Mindfulness practice has helped me take that next step in turning toward discomfort. It is a strong tool that I use to meet anger, frustration, sadness, and depression head on, no longer running away. I learned about "coming home" to a body I had spent most of my life hating. As I learn to listen to my body's sensations and experiences, I learn that cravings are just thoughts, and that they can pass THROUGH my busy mind IF I don't get hung up on them. I work with the space **between** my thoughts and behaviors, noticing that in that space is opportunity for a different response...a new way. In that space there is peace. This is the difference between reacting and responding. When I was IN the disease of compulsive overeating, I was in a constant state of reaction to the stimuli around and within me. Feeling happy? Eat. Feeling sad? Eat. Feeling confused? Eat. Feeling stressed? Definitely eat—make it sugary-sweet and crunchy and keep it coming! There is an acronym I use that really helps me, it's called HALT: never get too Hungry, Angry, Lonely, or Tired. Over the years I have added Elated and Depressed and now refer to it as HALTED. When I'm lost in these emotional states, I struggle to find the space between. I can get caught up in trying to make the 'negative' feelings go away (aversion) OR the 'positive' ones last forever (clinging).

Fast forward 8 years: I'm an active, joyful, mostly clear minded 51 year old woman. I absolutely love teaching Yoga, Pilates, Mindfulness, and Resiliency. Each morning, I commit to living mindfully and heartfully. I seek moderation in all things—except refined sugars from which I still abstain. I continue to maintain a 90 lb weight loss one breath at a time, trying never to take for granted the life I continue to discover one mindful step at a time.

Like many folks who discover dis-ease in their lives, it has been BECAUSE of my struggles with food, weight, and body image that I have discovered the richness of life. I don't say it brought me back to my life, as I didn't feel familiar with this way of living life. This is the life I was born to live—numbing myself with food began at such a young age I never had a chance to get to know who I was until now. I practice gratitude daily for this.

If this story is to be useful, there are a few things about which I want to be very clear. This is NOT about going on a diet. It is not about taking more control; it is about letting go. It is an exceptionally different orientation to health and weight, and so a big part of a mindful approach to eating is to begin to learn to find comfort in discomfort.

I ate compulsively to sooth feelings I called uncomfortable. Now, rather than trying to sooth them, I notice, allow, and accept that they are there (remember, this is NOT about making feelings go away, that would be control again). I take a slow deep breath and remind myself that feelings will pass IF I am willing to let them. Thoughts are just thoughts, they are not actions. And I take another breath...

"I have just three things to teach: simplicity, patience, compassion.
These three are your greatest treasures"

~ Lao Tzu

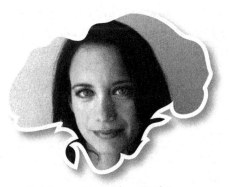

Marisol Oliva

Certified Integrative Nutrition Health Coach, Self-Love Coach

A weight-loss expert using a "no calorie counting" approach. Marisol is now working at Waistline Clinic.

I was born into a family of 5 kids, being a twin myself, in a small city north of Mexico just at the border of the United States. I love the outdoors and ever since I can remember, I have been interested in Mother Earth and learning how to protect her. Even at a young age, I truly believed we could find most of our answers in nature. At the age of 12, my dad passed away. It totally changed my life's perspective and I felt alone.

I started searching at this young age, for answers. I got interested in metaphysics, started learning about Universal Laws, past lives, invisible energy, subconscious mind, etc. I read a lot! I still do. Unfortunately there were no university careers that interested me, so I studied Business Administration and graduated 1rst in my generation. After that I did some Environmental Development studies.

I have always loved to read, and now it was food labels. I would spend hours at a grocery store just reading labels and deciding what was best for my body. I always knew that feeding my body any type of unnatural substance would harm me on the long run.

After having children, a new interested showed up. It had to do with our home environment and how it was affecting our children. I began learning about chemicals we breathe and put onto our bodies. By now people started coming up to me and asking me about my healthy eating and green living habits. So naturally I started my second career in Integrative Nutrition. After I was done studying, I found a new passion. Our gut and how healing it dramatically improves our health. I now teach people how they can repair their gut by feeding it the right prebiotics and probiotics and by eliminating foods that damage our intestines. I love to see how our bodies respond so amazingly after feeding it the nutrients it needs and leaving out as much toxins as we can. I can tell you, the answers do come from nature.

Contact Marisol:

✉ oliva_marisol@me.com

f facebook.com/Mi-Vida-Verde-por-Marisol-Oliva-756209667744856/timeline

in mx.linkedin.com/pub/marisol-oliva/ab/86/236

CHAPTER 24

WE *CAN* HEAL OURSELVES, EVEN ALLERGIES

By Marisol Oliva

I remember my mom having huge seasonal allergies every March. She had red swollen watery eyes, and she couldn't stop sneezing. I remember thinking to myself, "Is she exaggerating?" "Is she calling for attention?" Of course she wasn't, I just couldn't figure out why the "weather" had so much to do with her. Later on, I realized it was actually the wind carrying the pollen that was triggering her symptoms. This was a classic allergy outbreak.

With me, it started with skin allergies. My first recollection of it was when I was around six or seven years old. I remember my dad and I being outside our house where the sun could reach us. He would extend my arm under the sun and rub cortisol cream on my forearm then he'd do the next one. I still have brown spots there because of it. That's one of my earliest memories. Sometime after that, my allergies began to extend to behind my knees. They would itch soooo much! I actually preferred to experience pain than itching. I got to know my allergies so well. It would begin with a tiny white itchy dot on my skin, if I would scratch it, it would expand. Then there was the swelling! The white dot became red, swollen patches on my arms and legs. After a few days, and after applying some local medical cream, they would stop swelling. What was left was white, flaky skin, similar to dandruff. The heat did not help a bit, so no hot showers, and since I lived in a city where in summer the temperature would reach up to 50 °C, I was in trouble.

In my teens, I would have these itchy patches on my head and my eyebrows. I remember always having to apply cortisol. My mom then decided to take me to a skin doctor, a dermatologist. He did a tiny

177

surgery to take a piece of skin out from the back of my arm so they could test it. When we got the results a few days later, it just said "chronic dermatitis." What was that? It meant that I had a chronic case of something in my dermis (skin). Oh, that helped! So I had no clue whatsoever to what was wrong for years. As I grew up and was studying at college, I especially remember a very, very bad summer. It was the worst one ever! I had these red, swollen patches all over my arms. They were so big that it actually occurred to me the possibility of not being able to wear short sleeves ever again. I couldn't stand looking at my arms; I thought I would never go back to having normal skin ever. I was desperate, hopeless, and embarrassed. What was happening to me? Why wasn't my twin sister or anyone in my family suffering the same thing I was? Even though we were born prematurely and I stayed at the hospital for a whole month because of my weight, I still didn't understand. I tried every type of lotion out there. Some "natural" ones would itch, others would burn my skin, and others would make my skin even redder than it was and so on. I became a pro at recognizing the first sign of a coming flare and what type of cream to put on and at what stage. I had a short list of the only creams my skin could manage; the sad part is that most of them would contain some kind of medicine. At that time, I didn't care as long as the patches and itching were in control.

My mom kept telling me that my allergic flares would show up because of stress and every time I was nervous. She even suggested I take anxiety pills to control my nerves. I never took a pill for my allergies; I have never liked taking medicine.

In my late twenties, I moved to Mexico City where the weather is nice and somewhat cooler year round. By this time I had read many medical documents, books, magazines, and searched the Internet to find out what I had. According to my symptoms, I had eczema, which is a kind of allergy. I began noticing that after I had some specific kind of food, I would begin to feel the itchiness coming back right away. Now that I knew this came from living a certain lifestyle and from eating certain kinds of foods, I began to journal. I did this so I would know which foods I was allergic to. Some foods I was allergic to were: cucumber and tomato seeds, peaches, and chamomile, among others. The journaling exercise did help a lot. I kept a record of almost everything I ate differently than my regular diet. I felt like an investigator investigating a mystery, writing every little thing down. Even though this helped, the allergies weren't going away, so I decided to go to an allergist. I went a couple of times and did some blood tests, but they wanted me to go on a strict diet. They suggested no eggs, dairy, breads, and some fruits. I stopped going; that was essentially my diet and at that age I didn't know any other kind of foods to replace them with. The nice part is that I started reading every food label, so I could know what I was putting into my body, and I haven't stopped doing it. I still spend hours at the supermarket getting to know every little ingredient there is. I changed my diet to a healthier one (at my own pace), and I got healthier too, thankfully. I read every nutrition book I could. I read every medical and holistic healing website I could find. I was finally connecting all the pieces together.

I got married at age 30, and when I got pregnant, things started to change in my body. I began having allergies again, even after the baby was born. I don't know exactly what changed, I don't know if it was the hormones or just the fact that I had a baby inside. The allergies spread all over my eyes; sometimes I couldn't even open them when I woke up because of how swollen and puffy they were. It didn't just stop there; my neck was also very red, itchy and swollen. Little by little after journaling, I came to realize that cats caused me to have allergic reactions, so did perfumes and anything with harsh chemicals in them. I wanted to go natural, and the only way I could was avoiding the things that gave me flares.

Things got real bad especially when my husband and I would travel. I had allergic flares during every trip. I would have red swollen eyes, face, and neck in every picture. I couldn't put any make-up on my face and I had to travel with my special cream kit anywhere I went. I wrote down every possible culprit, the paper towels behind you at your seat on the plane, the hand soap in the bathroom, the harsh detergents or fabric softener on the plane blanket, etc. My mom would insist once again that it was my nerves. "Mom," I would tell her, "I really don't get nervous when I travel, my husband takes care of everything, I just pack the bags and that's it." So once again, I dismissed her possible conclusions.

But our last trip to Hong Kong was different. It got so bad that while we were at a mall, I saw an outside sign for a doctor. I knew I had to go inside. It was good of me to trust my intuition because once the Chinese doctor touched my wrists for five minutes he knew exactly what I was allergic to: chamomile and mint. Yes, mint! It just so happens that *every* time my husband and I would travel, he would offer me a stick of gum. That was the big mystery—the spearmint gum. But the most amazing thing was that the Chinese doctor knew exactly what was going on with me just by touching my wrists for five minutes. Oh my, I really wish Western medicine were this fast and successful without prescribing so many medicines. He also told me I was expecting, and I was. I was pregnant with my twins. I drank some herbs he gave me with water; they tasted awful, but I didn't mind. I was so happy. I never again had any mint and never again had any trouble when I traveled. Of course that didn't cure me but at least I knew what to avoid. I no longer had skin allergies, but my stomach became bloated quite often.

A new mystery began. Even though I was eating healthier, like more vegetables, more salads, more raw foods, green drinks, organic eggs, organic meats (but less of them), more wild caught fish, a little less dairy, incorporating super foods, avoiding GMO's, etc., I have always had a sweet tooth. Even though I switched to chocolate's darker versions, chocolate has been my weak side. When I go out with friends or family or any kind of gatherings, if there is cake, cookies, or brownies, I will eat some. I don't drink alcohol and have never smoked, but I do love sugar. That was a huge problem in my life because I later learned that it was feeding the Candida yeast, and every time I had a vaginal yeast infection, my gynecologist would recommend I take antibiotics. I didn't know it at that time but every time I had antibiotics, they would destroy and unbalance my intestinal microflora. Antibiotics kill bad microorganisms, but sadly, they also kill the good ones. We need those good microorganisms to help us digest our foods and help our intestines absorb the nutrients in our foods. What did my allergies have to do with this? Well actually, quite a lot! The antibiotics would create permeability in my intestines, meaning I was having a leaky gut. Actual holes in my intestines where large food particles would penetrate my blood system. My immune system would go crazy destroying itself, thinking these large food particles were "invaders." This war was causing the inflammation in my body, my skin, and now, my stomach. Yet no doctor ever told me to take the antibiotics with caution or ever suggested I take probiotics afterwards. Not one! I had to learn about gut health and about probiotics (the good bacteria) by myself, again by reading. The good thing is that I have always loved to read.

So it's of utmost importance that we pay attention to our gut health. It's actually our second brain, and it is 80% of our immune system. Unfortunately, it's not as easy as taking a handful of probiotic pills every day. It's much more than that; it is stopping the triggers in their tracks. A good place to start is by doing an elimination diet. It also helps to detox the body and help it to eliminate the accumulated toxins, so that you can give it a chance to work at its optimal level. It's very important to take the right kind of probiotic supplements, especially natural probiotics found in fermented foods like cultured vegetables, kombucha, and kefir, among others. It's giving your intestines a way to repair themselves so your body *can* actually heal itself. And it's crucial to provide for your body the nutrients it needs by eating whole foods such as green and cruciferous vegetables, grass-fed organic meats and organic eggs, healthy fats like olive oil, avocados, coconut, and by avoiding genetically modified oils. You should also eat wild caught fish, nuts, and seeds. Limit your sugar intake such as simple carbohydrates and simple sugars, especially high fructose corn syrup or fructose in general. Remember, it doesn't matter if you eat huge amounts of healthy foods if your intestines aren't absorbing the nutrients in them.

As for me, I took my last antibiotic for the last yeast infection I had in early January 2012. Because of the antibiotics, by February of that same year, I became allergic to strawberries and artificial vitamin C. I had red, swollen eyelids for almost two months. But now, I knew better: I stayed away from sugar, I knew which topical creams to use, which probiotic supplements to take. I had kefir for breakfast and had kombucha drinks often. The allergy eventually disappeared without any medical treatment. Since then, I haven't had any allergic outbreaks and, of course, I haven't had any antibiotics, artificial sweeteners, and only small amounts of gluten, dairy, sugar, and

GMOs. I can tell you that the foods that come from Mother Nature healed me along with my extraordinarily intelligent body (which we all have); we just have to learn to listen to it.

My last recommendation, apart from restoring your gut, is to live a peaceful and happy life with as little stress as possible. Go follow your passions; it's what the Universe intended for you.

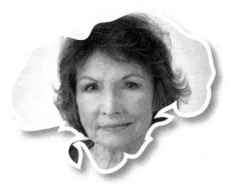

Marsha Mendizza

Marsha knows what it means to lose and reclaim her life.

She was at the top of her game when stricken with Chronic Fatigue Syndrome/Fibromyalgia, a debilitating, misunderstood condition.

She was distinguished as an educator, developing training programs for the State of California, Department of Education and designed educational programs nationally for the United Centers for Spiritual Living. She co-trained The Centering Lab for the prestigious National Training Labs Institute for Applied Behavioral Science for 17 years.

Her private practice as a counselor/coach thrived.

Then she got sick; lost her marriage, work, and the ability to think, or move without pain. Depression replaced optimism. Her life as she knew it was over.

Traditional medicine failed her; nine years passed without a diagnosis, treatment, or relief.

Then she discovered integrative medicine, and began her journey back to vitality.

She is grounded in the benefits and limitations of traditional medicine, TCM, homeopathy, Ayurveda, osteopathy, nutritional medicine, movement, brain restoration and the new field of genetic medicine.

Today she is energetic, creative, highly functioning and passionate about assisting others reclaim their own lives. Marsha knows that *"Healing is not a one size fits all project", and* tailors her consultation to the individual needs, strengths and weakness of each client to restore physical, emotional, creative wellbeing.

"This illness was a gift demanding I activate my best self to heal. My greatest satisfaction is in helping others mobilize their own innate capacity to overcome inner & outer obstacles, and thrive."

Contact Marsha:

www.marshamendizza.com

📞 **Mobile: (818)427-5680**

📞 **Office: (818)782-8533**

✉️ **marsha@marshamendizza.com**

📘 **facebook.com/mmendizza**

🐦 **@MMendizza**

📇 **linkedin.com/pub/marsha-mendizza/a/951/286**

CHAPTER 25

LIFE, INTERRUPTED

By Marsha Mendizza

It was a special Monday morning, so I dressed up. A new silk blouse caressed my skin under a crisp teal suit. Impeccable make-up, great hair, a Hobo bag slung over one shoulder symbolized a purposeful happiness as I slipped into my favorite shoes and strode confidently out the door.

Even LA traffic was easy driving to the office. I was excited. I won raises for my staff in grinding budget negotiations with a tough CFO. I couldn't wait to break the good news.

Even better, Saturday night my husband and I celebrated our one year wedding anniversary. Smart, sexy, funny, handsome, w-a-y upwardly mobile, Jim was a dream man. We vowed to love each other all our lives. My white gold wedding ring set with a fiery opal sparkled in the morning sun. I loved and was loved. My heart was full. Life was wonderful.

For the millionth time I glanced down at my ring, and suddenly, a wave of dizziness swept over me. I gripped the wheel tightly and focused hard to avoid hitting the next car.

The dizziness passed, but my stomach churned as I walked into the office at nine and celebrated with my work family, smiling through slightly clenched teeth, trying not to throw up.

At ten, in the middle of a meeting, I felt another wave come over me, this one severed my brain-mouth connection leaving me so fatigued I was mildly incoherent. I escaped to the bathroom, my blouse now sticking to clammy skin. I had to hold onto the wall to keep my balance as I walked back to the office.

What is going on here?

The flu. I must have the flu… or maybe food poisoning. I called Jim… maybe he has it too. "I feel fine, honey. Just great! See you tonight. Love you."

At 11:30 I called it and went home, barely able to drive; soaked with sweat, I crawled into bed.

I never went back to the office, my professional home for seven years.

BODY ON FIRE

The next morning, the strain of lifting a cup of tea produced hot pain. At first only the muscles needed to lift the cup—hand, wrist, arm, shoulder—hurt. Soon, all the muscles in my body were on fire. The flu on steroids.

A low-grade fever accompanied "brain fog." I left one room and walked feebly into another, and upon arrival would have no idea whatsoever why I was there. Random episodes of vertigo and constant exhaustion transformed me into a stooped over, frail creature.

My digestion froze. Not much could be assimilated.

After a week, I went to the doctor who promptly placed me on disability. "What's wrong with me?" "Burnout," he said and told me to rest.

I rested for a month and was still completely exhausted. I went to another doctor who suggested anti-depressants, which I declined. (Like, of course I was depressed! Depression was a side effect of something else!) I went to another doctor who prescribed a walk on the beach and an ice cream cone.

Jim was empathic, supportive, and sympathetic for the first year as we went to doctor after doctor after doctor with no help. He made my breakfast then went to work. After work he made my dinner and walked me to the couch where I usually fell asleep watching mind-numbing TV.

I kept going to doctors with Jim, and then alone after he divorced me. A year after our first anniversary, he was through. He didn't sign up for this.

I was moved into a one-bedroom apartment in Van Nuys, and he left.

Every day for the next 8 years, I woke up hoping, praying that today would be better, and every day it felt as though all the cells in my body had lead weights tied to them. All I really wanted to do was lie down. Anywhere.

I had lost my brain, work, and marriage. I still had a body, but she had betrayed me and was only a source of fatigue and pain.

But I never lost the intention that someday, somehow, I would recover my life.

KEEPING THE FAITH

These two truths helped me keep the faith:

"The unconscious always tries to produce an impossible situation in order to force the individual to bring out his very best. Otherwise one stops short of one's best, one is not complete, one does not realize oneself."

C. J. Jung

My situation was impossible. I vowed to do my best, keep the faith, and hold on.

And from the I Ching:

"The Turning Point: After a time of decay comes the turning point. The powerful light that has been banished returns."

I kept the faith that light would return and held on.

HEALING

And then one day I began to heal.

Nine years later, on another Monday, I went to the next doctor on my list. Ninety minutes later, I was weeping with relief because I was given not one, but two diagnoses:

"Chronic fatigue and immune dysfunction syndrome (CFIDS) is a debilitating and complex disorder characterized by profound fatigue; Fibromyalgia is a disorder characterized by widespread musculoskeletal pain accompanied by fatigue, sleep, memory and mood issues." — Mayo Clinic.

There was (and is) no known cause or cure; no magic bullet.

Naming my condition was a critical turning point. I was not crazy, my condition was not "all in my head," nor the "yuppie flu," accusations thrust on me by those who didn't understand and were sick and tired of me being sick and tired.

My healing began.

ILLNESS AS A TEACHER

Fundamental to transforming illness into restored vitality was the (reluctant) acceptance that my illness was not my enemy, but my greatest teacher. I had not been victimized by fate; I had been challenged to learn something, including why I got sick, and how to not just recover but to thrive.

First lesson: All my life I had driven my body like a machine. An acupuncturist stated it more clearly:

"You are Not a Toyota!" My body possesses great wisdom and had responded intelligently by collapsing when I drove myself too hard. I reframed how I identified myself: I am a spiritual, emotional, mental, and physical human being. My learning was to always include a check-in with my "physical self" in the morning when making decisions about how I used my day.

This breaking news, ironically, gave me power. I realized that if my body was smart enough to say "no" to being assaulted, she was also smart enough to say "yes" to being supported. I remembered another quote of Jung: "There is a natural gradient towards wholeness within every individual." I made a decision to trust my body's intelligence and to support her in every way I could.

Second lesson: I learned the psychological, environmental, and biological conditions that made me sick and the remedies that made me well. This took a bunch of years.

Here are a few of them, which are not confined only to my illness, but address the origins of disease in general. These learnings have been distilled over two decades from Homeopathy, Traditional Chinese Medicine, Integrative Medicine, Ayurveda, Osteopathy, Genetic Medicine, Neuroscience, Food as Medicine, and Jungian Psychoanalysis.

The digestive system—this is the root of all disease and all health. I spent years restoring my "digestive fire." Nobody can function optimally unless the digestive system works. One easy reference is: http://gapsdiet.com, a possible substitute for the shelves of antacid remedies at your local pharmacy. (Just go into your pharmacy and look at them! Amazing!)

Nutrients—the job of our digestive system is to deliver nutrients to our cells. If they don't receive the nutrients they need, the body will decline. An organic diet is essential—pesticides are bad.

My gut was severely compromised by a lifetime of substituting nutrients with processed foods, sugar, including grain-based carbohydrates that metabolized as sugar, combined with an overuse of antibiotics in my early life, mercury from amalgam fillings and lead from auto exhaust, creating an acidic "biological terrain", a happy environment for infection. The beginning of my healing was in my gut. It's unbelievable that a very smart adult woman didn't know how to eat. A Nutritional Therapy Association practitioner was very helpful in teaching me how to eat (http://nutritionaltherapy.com/).

First, I needed food. Then, supplementation, based on sound testing, both clinical and applied kinesiology.

Battling infection—with the lack of nutrients and the presence of mercury and lead, my body developed chronic subclinical (under the clinical radar) and clinical bacterial and viral infections. (Initially, CFIDS was thought to be caused by the Epstein-Barr virus.) I had the amalgams that had been poisoning my system for decades removed from my teeth. No other way. Inconvenient, expensive…necessary. Bottom line: When my cells were nourished and my body was strengthened, I had fewer infections

Neurotransmitter imbalance—because my gut, sometimes called the "second brain," was compromised, over time the balance in my actual brain was also compromised. (Of course I was depressed!). In addition to restoring my digestive fire, I also restored the balance in my brain with biofeedback and amino acid protocols.

CHOCOLATE BREAK

How are you doing so far? Sound complicated, hard, impossible? Want to stop reading and eat chocolate?

I totally get it.

TRAP

When I began to really understand what it would take to get well, I didn't think I could do it. Too expensive, too complicated, too hard: "I just can't do this."

This was a trap that I almost fell into… like just wanting to go to bed forever is a trap. With help, I avoided this life-stealing trap, kept the faith, and moved on.

THERAPY

Remember what Jung said about the unconscious producing an impossible situation? I entered therapy and uncovered the psychological causes of my illness.

TREATMENT

I learned that a lifestyle change and psychotherapy wasn't enough. I needed treatment, and specific kinds of treatment. These are just a few of the approaches that have generated increasing vitality and health.

Integrative Medicine—While most MDs were unable to help me, I found an Integrative Medicine MD (a term being used more frequently to replace both "Alternative" and '"Complementary" Medicine) who could. MDs can run blood tests and have valuable and proven clinical treatments that helped me to heal. Just because some traditional doctors couldn't help, I discovered some who could. Integrative Medicine is good medicine.

Energetic Medicine—I found acupuncture helpful at the beginning but insufficient for complete healing. Homeopathy strengthens the entire person at all levels. It is subtle, powerful healing. I will use homeopathic remedies for the rest of my life.

Genetic Medicine—This fast-growing specialty is being incorporated by more doctors. The effect of all other modalities and healing approaches will be reduced unless and until any genetic weaknesses in the body are restored to full functioning. Because I'm committed to total health and vitality for the rest of my life, I ordered a simple test from https://www.23andme.com. For $99, I received the information about certain genetic mutations or "speed bumps" that I was born with that inhibit optimal health, and I have a protocol to restore my "methylation pathways" which is producing even more vitality than I could have ever imagined. It is very exciting.

Today, I have not only recovered but am thriving. It became clear to me that the key elements of my healing journey can benefit others, each in his or her own way. Today, through my counseling and coaching practice, I am helping others to heal and thrive.

It's true that while there is no one-size-fits-all, these key essentials that supported my healing may support yours.

- First: Find, then keep the faith, remembering that faith is the evidence of things unseen.

- Second: Your Illness/condition is your teacher. You are not a victim.

- Third: You are not a Toyota to just be driven. Your body is smarter than you or your illness. Listen!

- Fourth: Whether you are vibrantly healthy or ill, always remember that the gut is the beginning of your health or illness.

- Fifth: You may need treatment in addition to making a lifestyle change. Keep researching until you find the practitioner(s) right for you. You may need multiple approaches to your wellness.

- Sixth: Watch out for traps. Just because you want to lie down all the time doesn't mean you should. Move, both physically, mentally, and emotionally.

- Seventh: Find a good friend, family member, or therapist who will always be there for you, no matter how you feel.

- Eighth: Find the best therapist or coach to facilitate your restoration to health, both psychological and physical. Your healing depends on a cooperative strengthening of psyche, spirit, and body.

- Ninth: Always enjoy good chocolate, an essential food group.

I'm writing this on a Thursday. The day before me is rich with possibility. I am looking at my beautiful ring right now. The opal is my birthstone and sparkles as the sun reflects its fire. I designed this ring that once served as my wedding ring. Today, it is a symbol of the light that shines for all of us.

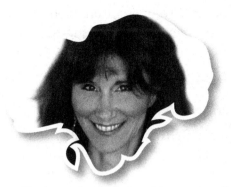

Dr. Ritamarie Loscalzo

Dr. Ritamarie Loscalzo is fiercely committed to transforming our current broken disease-care system into a true health care system where each and every practitioner is skilled at finding the root cause of health challenges and using ancient healing wisdom married with modern scientific research to restore balance.

As the founder of the Institute of Nutritional Endocrinology, Dr. Ritamarie specializes in using the wisdom of nature to restore balance to hormones with a special emphasis on thyroid, adrenal, and insulin imbalances. Her practitioner training programs empower health and nutrition practitioners to get to the root cause by using functional assessments and natural therapeutics to balance the endocrine system, the master controller.

Dr. Ritamarie is a licensed Doctor of Chiropractic with Certifications in Acupuncture, Nutrition, Herbal Medicine, and HeartMath®. She's also a certified living foods chef, instructor, and coach, and she has trained and certified hundreds of others in the art of using palate-pleasing whole fresh food as medicine.

A best-selling author, speaker, and internationally recognized nutrition and women's health authority with over 23 years of clinical experience, Dr. Ritamarie offers online courses, long-distance coaching and counseling, and deeply empowering and informative live events. Her wildly popular practitioner certification program empowers health and wellness professionals to unravel the mystery of their clients' complex health challenges, so they become known as go-to practitioners for true healing and lasting results.

Contact Dr. Ritamarie:

www.drritamarie.com/vibrant/presskit/

facebook.com/DrRitamarieLoscalzo

@DrRitamarie

CHAPTER 26

UNLOCKING MY INNER HEALER AND MY JOURNEY TO HEALTH AND JOY

By Dr. Ritamarie Loscalzo

Like most people just graduating college, I felt invincible. I was hired immediately out of college into a well-paid position with a well-known high tech company, and I felt elated.

After a job switch and a big promotion a year later, I was living in the fast lane. I drove long distances each day and ate lots of restaurant meals with clients, wining and dining on rich foods and even richer desserts.

Then, suddenly, I began to develop vague and uncomfortable symptoms.

I had a constant post-nasal drip and sinus congestion and was put on steroid injections and antibiotics. I was told I needed to have cryosurgery to freeze the tissue in my sinuses to make them stop dripping. I started getting headaches again. When I was a college student, the headaches were unbearable, and I was prescribed valium to control them. That made it so I couldn't get out of bed in the morning, so I stopped and reverted to aspirin. So when the headaches started again, I began to take aspirin, sometimes several times a day.

After that, I developed severe burning stomach pain and went to the doctor for an evaluation. They put me on ulcer medication, told me to drink lots of milk, and referred me to a gastroenterologist to test to see if I indeed had an ulcer.

In the meantime, I was suffering from almost constant fogginess and an inability to focus. I called it brain fog. I would be talking to people and have to concentrate really hard to understand what they were saying.

I did the invasive ulcer testing, requiring me to swallow barium and be scoped. The results were negative. The day the gastroenterologist sat me down with the "good news" that I didn't have an ulcer was the turning point in my life. I replied, "Great! So what's causing the pain?" His answer forever changed my life. He replied, "We don't know so just keep taking the ulcer medication and drinking lots of milk."

I was devastated. "For how long? " I asked. "For as long as you need to, maybe forever," was the reply. At that moment the vision of me in a wheelchair on dialysis at age 50 bounced through my brain. If this was life at 25, what would I be like at 50 if I didn't find the cause and correct it?

Then I asked the fated question, likely divinely inspired, "Could it be my diet?"

"Of course not. Diet doesn't have anything to do with it."

I was challenged. Challenged to find a solution for my current discomforts and for whatever lies in my future. I was determined to feel well again.

Intrigued by the thought that it might be my diet, I went to the public library and checked out as many books as I could find on nutrition. I read Carlton Fredericks, Adele Davis, and other popular nutrition authors of the time. Back in the 1980's we didn't have the internet to search!

I started drinking more milk, skim milk as that was what was suggested. I threw away the white flour products and exchanged them for whole wheat bread. I started eating more fresh vegetables. I started to exercise regularly, taking up running.

Overall, there was some improvement but only intermittently. I had a couple of good days here and there mixed in with the bad days, instead of just bad days.

I bought *The 5 Day Allergy Relief System* book and fasted for five days to remove all allergens. I felt fantastic when I fasted, but as soon as I began to eat again, the fog and headaches returned. On the good days I was excited, happy, focused, and pain free. On the bad days I was achy, exhausted, and in a fog. I felt frustrated. Overwhelmed and defeated.

I found a doctor at a center called the "Medical Nutrition Center," and she taught me about gut bacteria and its importance in health. She assessed that I had an overgrowth of candida albicans, a type of fungus, and many food allergies. I began to take supplements—lots of them—and a prescription anti-fungal medication called Nystatin.

She advised I stop consuming all alcohol, sugar, bread, and caffeine. Wow. What's left to eat?

I did exactly what she said and the number of good days started to become more frequent, perhaps up to a few days a week. I felt so good on the good days that I became more and more determined. I took meticulous notes of everything I ate and how I felt. Likely, they are still buried in a drawer somewhere. I was frustrated, hopeful, and very determined. I knew there were answers, and eventually, I found my way to true healing.

I was sitting at a service station, waiting for my oil to be changed, reading a book about health.

A man sat down beside me and asked about my reading material, inquiring about my health. Then he recommended a book that would forever change my life—and perhaps has changed and even saved thousands of other lives. The book was called *Fasting Can Save Your Life*, by Dr. Herbert Shelton. It sounded odd, but I was curious so I bought it. The book was very different from any other book I had ever read. It talked about toxicity as the underlying cause of all disease, then went on to describe all the effects of overwhelming our body's ability to eliminate toxins.

I felt as if Dr. Shelton were describing my life up until the point when my health starting failing me. I'd been eating processed food, lots of sugar and caffeine, and oxidized fats. We used toxic cleaning products in our home and lived in fear and worry about being able to make ends meet. All the negative diet and lifestyle factors Dr. Shelton described in the book were those I'd grown up on. Most of the contributors to optimal health were missing for me.

My mysterious savior at the service station also gave me the name of a nearby retreat center that ascribed to the teachings in the book. After finishing the book, I arranged for my now-husband and I to visit and check it out. I was entranced, and wanted to check myself in immediately. Unfortunately there was this little issue of...my job!

I lay awake at night trying to figure out how I could get four weeks off work so I could participate in a cleanse.

As luck (or divine intervention) would have it, I landed in the hospital with emergency surgery for an ectopic (tubal) pregnancy. And when the surgeon said I would need a six week leave from work to recuperate, I knew I'd been given my chance.

I checked into what was called the Religious School of Natural Hygiene and began an extended water fast.

As my body shrunk, my mind cleared and my energy soared. I spent my days reading, listening to tapes, and writing notes of forgiveness to many people who'd wronged me. I sent notes of apology to people I'd wronged. I was in bed by 9 pm and slept until 6 am. The stress of my job was behind me as I focused my attention on one thing and one thing alone—my healing.

My family thought I was completely nuts and feared for my life. I went from 115 to 92 pounds in 28 days. I looked like a skeleton, yet I'd never felt better in my life. I made a vow to continue to only nourish myself with the foods my body would thrive on. I vowed that sugar and processed food would never again pass through my lips. I learned new ways to prepare food using only whole fresh plant ingredients. And I made a decision to quit my job and go back to school to become a doctor so I could teach people how to embrace and unleash their natural healing powers –and to do it with much more ease than I had.

After leaving the retreat center, I enrolled in some anatomy and physiology classes at the local community college to see if I had enough interest and aptitude to succeed. I instantly fell in love with my studies.

I quit my job in the spring, got married in the early summer, and got certified as a massage therapist so I could create some income while I studied. In the autumn of the following year, 1987, I enrolled in chiropractic school and, shortly thereafter, found a long distance nutrition master's degree program through the University of Bridgeport. I graduated in 1991 with two degrees—Doctor of Chiropractic and Master of Science in Human Nutrition.

The entire process, from my own healing in 1985 to getting my license and getting my thesis approved took almost seven years. The journey to actually regain my health took several years of trial and error, experimentation, and lots of time and money.

I managed to keep my excellent health and become even healthier throughout my studies by starting my day, every day, with at least a quart of blended greens, cycling to and from school whenever I could, and keeping a positive attitude. I "kept my eyes on the prize." I ate lots of salads and vegetables and taught myself to prepare foods in a whole new way. I found I had a knack for combining whole fresh foods in interesting ways and making dishes even my skeptical friends enjoyed. I had a few ups and downs as I experimented with the proportions of macronutrients that worked best for me, and I learned a lot about personalized nutrition planning.

I later went on to add acupuncture and herbal medicine to my repertoire and, even later, became certified in my absolute favorite system of managing and transforming stress, HeartMath! I now have a thriving business supporting thousands of people around the globe to make healthier choices and to balance their immune, endocrine, and digestive systems using foods, herbs, and the power of positive attitude, along with sunshine, sleep, movement, a clean environment, and lots of fun.

I feel healthier and more energetic now than I did back in my 20's. I still choose only whole fresh foods, have not touched processed foods or sugar since before my fast, and I teach others the art of creating delicious meals on a monthly internet show broadcast from my kitchen.

I believe we all have an inner healer, sometimes locked inside. Health is restored by unlocking our healer from the prison of a toxic environment, processed foods, toxic emotions, and a lack of vision and passion. I live each day in an attitude of gratitude for all I have and for the opportunity I had three decades ago to experience chronic ill health. Had I not made the changes I did back then, and continued with the lifestyle I had been leading, it's quite possible that I would not be here to write this. My dear mom left us prematurely at age 56. I am grateful to have been able to choose a different path and to be able to share my expertise and wisdom with others on their healing journeys.

And I am forever grateful for the un-named man in the gas station, the one who lives in my heart as the guardian angel who saved my life.

CHAPTER 27

SEEING HEALING IN A NEW LIGHT
By Tatjana Kulibabo

"The Wound is Where the Light Enters You"

-Rumi

Sometimes unexpected, cataclysmic events happen for which it seems that nothing in life has prepared you for but which somehow transform you and give your life deeper meaning. Sometimes these come in packages which thrill and inspire, sometimes they come in packages that can humble and terrify, but both seem to invite us to go deeper into this mystery that we call life.

Over ten years ago, one early autumn day, I received one of these life-transforming calling cards. I was living in Asia, in a training centre nestled between rice fields and forest, on the outskirts of a small, growing town. The late summer heat was waning, and the cooler days brought a sense of the coming changes of the fall. The tips of the leaves in the woods nearby were showing hints of the transformation to come. It began subtly, surreptitiously, but it was an event that initiated what continues to transform me. I noticed some blurriness, an odd feeling of a tiny blind spot when I was reading. I kept rubbing my eyes but to no avail. It must be tiredness, I thought, and left it, thinking some rest and a walk in the woods would help.

It had been a stressful few months leading up to this event, after all. I had been working long hours, sometimes 14 hour days. Most core shaking of all, a friend and mentor had committed suicide a month before. I was drowning in grief; I needed rest.

Over the next few days, I noticed blind spots in both eyes, which were now beginning to grow. The blurry spots became spots of darkness, like inkblots, and these inkblots grew over the next few days to occlude my entire field of vision. Everything I looked at was completely opaque, engulfed in this dark void that permitted nothing, no movement, no shadow. Not even light. Nothing.

I was not having blurry vision, or a few blind spots. I had gone blind in both eyes.

It was the most terrifying thing I had ever experienced. Without visual input—without the ability to recognize the faces of loved ones, to read, to be calmed by nature, to look at art—I had lost my inspirations and connections to the external world. I felt empty and lost, my inner world desolate, lifeless.

A flurry of activity followed. Tests, tests, more tests. Nothing was showing up. There was suspicion of MS, but admittedly, it was a severe and unusual presentation, so even that was in question. No diagnosis, so no treatment, just waiting. And then, unbelievably, as quietly and as surreptitiously as the blindness came on, it also went, and my vision was restored. Within a month, I could see again.

But this announced only the beginning.

Over the next 12 years, much unfolded. I took this event as a "sign" that I need to radically transform my life. I checked off destinations on my bucket list with wild abandon. I travelled voraciously. I interned with a Nobel Peace prize winner; I meditated in Burmese temples; I watched sunsets over the Himalayan Mountains. I went to fasting retreats, did detoxes, changed my diet, studied yoga and Qi gong, changed my lifestyle. I changed countries of residence a few times. I met a Traditional Chinese doctor whose treatments and teachings inspired me to take up a new path. I started to change careers.

On some level, I thought that all of this earned me some protection from whatever had brought my health crisis on. Like collecting points to earn favor with God.

But, as it turned out, these changes were not enough. Life wanted me to go deeper, because within that same time period I also had more episodes: of blindness, an inability to walk, to use my hands, to eat, or to speak. I had episodes multiple times. Several diagnoses rolled in, but years after the first onset, the majority vote went to Relapsing Remitting Multiple Sclerosis.

I remember coming back from the hospital, calling my father, and letting him know of the diagnosis. He paused for a moment and then said something I will always remember and think of often: "Never forget that you can heal yourself."

My father's encouraging words kept my spirits high, kept me moving forward with positive changes. But the cloud of doubt within me was growing stronger and this doubt undermined the changes I was making. I could not anchor them and quickly would fall into old habits once my health was more stable. I doubted. Was it possible to heal from this illness? Why were there not more stories of people healing from MS? There were some, but by now, the cloud of doubt had grown so I doubted even them.

Healing from illness can be a demanding journey — not only my body but my mind and my faith in my ability to heal were being weakened. I decided I needed to pack well for this trip, as I entered this holy labyrinth of healing.

REGAINING TRUST THAT OUR BODIES CAN HEAL

In the beginning, diagnoses, fears, and projections of these into the future dominated the underground currents of my mental landscape. In the beginning, I didn't quite know where to start to regain trust that my body can heal, so I started with what I could see in the world around me, in nature.

I realized that everywhere I look on this planet I can see life growing in unexpected, inhospitable places. One of my favorite examples: the Welwithchia plant of the great deserts of Namibia — deserts so arid that virtually no rainfall graces them for years, yet the plants can survive on just the coastal sea fogs alone.

No less amazing nor miraculous are more common sights, such as plants fighting their way through concrete walls and roads, somehow finding a place for themselves and surviving in and amidst unforgiving life denying concrete. The little plant that fights its way through the crack in the sidewalk is an everyday miracle, a testament to the primacy of life.

Everywhere I look, life wants to live. Life wants to thrive. I decided to access in me that which was in that little plant fighting through the concrete and in those amazing plants in the desert.

I realized our bodies house miracles. Hundreds of thousands of biochemical and electrical reactions happen in our cells every second; there is intelligence that courses through every cell of our being down to the fundamental building blocks of life, our DNA, which has the capacity of self repair. The fact that if I cut my finger, it will heal on its own—this does not cease to amaze me. Despite the fact that many things can go wrong, it is undeniable that many more things go right, and we are in fact walking and living miracles, hardwired to heal. We are that way, capable of healing and self repair, just by virtue of being alive.

I decided to access the will to live and the will to heal.

As the beautiful teachings of Carolyn Myss have taught me, one of the most important questions I can ask myself is not how to heal, but why. Why do I want to heal? What about my life is worth living? What about my life is worth celebrating each and every day? I started with small reasons, small joys, small gratitudes in the times that were darkest, hardest, where I could not give a bigger answer or much of an answer at all—these were my saving graces. And they built momentum until this determination drove my healing. Deeply, consciously aware that I wanted to affirm life.

I thought back to the numbers and statistics I had heard when I was first told I had MS. Statistics that were daunting and haunted me. And I thought: "So what? That is a story about the past, and it might even be a story that is skewed or even false. The present moment is the only place from which we have possibility, the only place that is real. It is the only thing worth focusing on because it's the only place from which change can happen. And if of all the little plants that try to fight their way through the sidewalk, even if only one out of a million succeed, why can't I be that one in a million too?" I have so much love and respect for those little plants, and wherever I see them I thank them, I bless them.

THINKING OF ILLNESS WITH A NEW AWARENESS

Illness can also be a failed attempt to heal you. I read an article in a medical journal recently on the need to revise our paradigms with respect to disease—this article specifically dealt with cancer. In it, cancer is not presented as an enemy that is trying to destroy us, but rather, as a failed *mechanism of wound repair.* When the underlying wound stimulus (physical or psychological) was addressed, cancer was shown to go into complete remission, even in metastasis. Of course, the physical results of this failure can be dangerous and need to be addressed, but the underlying point is deeply thought provoking. I couldn't help but wonder: Can other illnesses be viewed as a failed attempt to heal you? An attempt that lost its way but nonetheless that points you in the direction of healing, of deeper truths, deeper healing?

It is also true, as Carolyn Myss writes, that it might turn out sometimes in healing that our body does not heal but that our spirit does. This too is healing.

A few months ago, I gave a presentation in Qatar on the role of nutrition and the microbiome in the healing of autoimmune diseases to an audience of MS Society members, doctors, and pharmacy reps. I was blessed to have my friend and passionate medical professional Dr. Maral Yazdandoost join me to give an engaging and informative talk on methods of stress reduction.

I was taken by the paradigm shift that is happening, the molecular biology revolution that is radically revising what we know about autoimmunity, and I was taken by the insight that healing our gut can heal autoimmune conditions. Before the talk, a woman in a wheelchair came up to the table where I was sitting and asked if she could join me. I was immediately at ease with this warm, gentle-hearted, soft-spoken woman. She had had MS for about 30 years, and as we spoke she said, "Why should I be unhappy that I have MS? God has chosen me as a special one. I have been given a gift. Through this illness in this lifetime, I can cleanse my spirit of all of its impurities. This is a great blessing. "

And as we talked, my spirit stood still. She spoke of a deeply resonating truth. Yes, there are many different ways and angles to look at healing, at what it takes, at what we need, at what it is. In the beginning, I looked eagerly to the experiences of others: What worked for them? What helped them? How can it help me? I still place much value on the community for learning and healing, but I also can see that at the bottom all of our journeys are exquisitely unique, and the starting place for the discovery of these answers lies in our own stories, hearts, and spirits.

Yes, it's true. This has been a gift. An odd gift, an unexpected gift, many times a rejected but persistently returning gift, a painful gift, a heart wrenching gift, but a heart and spirit opening gift, a love bearing gift, a soul redemptive gift. I am not "healed," but I am healing, moving in the right direction. And right now, to me, this is what matters.

Conclusion

My mom passed away 5 years ago from cancer. Amongst other things, she also had Celiac disease, which had only been diagnosed after she had suffered with it for 30 years.

"When I reflect on all I know now, I could have helped my mom and maybe she'd still be with us today" I said to my husband. But before I had even finished my sentence, I already knew the answer; she would never have listened to me.....then the sadness settled in my heart!

Why am I sharing this very personal story with you? Because now that you've read all these wonderful testimonials, now that all these people have shared with you not only their pain but also their joy in finding alternative solutions, what are you going to do? You see, all this is only as good as what you intend to do with it. Other treatment methods exist out there, that I can promise you. No matter what the media are saying, no matter what your brother, sister or anyone is saying....it does exist for those who are looking for it.

Now that being said, I'm not suggesting that you should stop any treatment or regime you are currently following through your doctor because the truth is that you shouldn't! Not for now at least. And don't forget to keep your doctor in the know about everything you're doing. But at the same time, check it out and see for yourself; investigate, research.... after all, it's your body, your health and your life!

This book is already a great starting point. You will get inspiration, you will get the proof that it is possible. In some instances you will even get some ideas, little steps that you can implement right now where you are, without having to spend a fortune or without having to change everything in your life just yet. However, I can also make you another promise. If you do take on board even a third of what has been shared with you within the pages of this book, you will change everything in your life!

I know this for a fact because there is no stronger force than that of being healthy.

Once you start feeling better you will realize that what you are doing is actually working, that you do indeed have the power to recover your health, that you are the captain of your own ship. And let me tell you, there is nothing more encouraging and inspiring than that. Then, once you can see that you are getting better, something else will happen; you'll start to trust yourself and your decisions, so guess what? You'll make more decisions related to your health and you'll never stop! This is how you change your life completely.

Both I and the entire Crazy Broccoli team wish you fantastic health for the future.

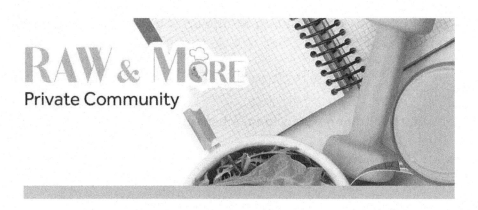

RAW & MORE
Private Community

We all want Shakira's waistline and the athletic silhouette of Cameron Diaz but what else can you do when no matter what you try....it just doesn't go away? You watch your portion size, you count calories, you spend all your free time at the gym, yet still nothing works. The inches aren't budging, you can't just melt them away. So what now?

Allergies can cause many symptoms and feeling bloated or overweight are 2 of the main ones.

If you have food sensitivity, you have an inflammation and if you do, then your belly won't go away through diet and exercise alone. You need a full reset and that's just what I do.

Getting the body of your dreams may be one of the most difficult goals to achieve. Why? Because everything you may have heard so far is wrong and, worst case scenario, if you've already tried a few diets before it probably made your situation even worse.

There is a reason why the pounds don't leave your waist and that reason has nothing to do with your genes. It has everything to do with what you eat, when you eat and most importantly how well you digest your food.

In order to help other women regain control over their own body and feel healthy and sexy inside and out, I've developed a special platform where I share cutting-edge information, special recipes, exercise routines, amazing interviews with leaders in the industry, monthly seminars on specific subjects and a Q & A call along with access to a private community to support you so you are never alone in this journey.

Don't delay any longer….solutions do exist so let me help you become the REAL YOU!

www.rawandmoremag.com/membership

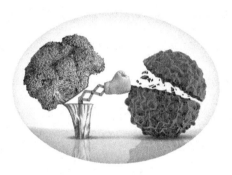

The End